Enoch Merlyn

Reclaiming Calm

Life Strategies for Today's Anxious Generation

Praise the Lord

First edition

Introduction 5
Chapter 1: Understanding the Storm 10
Chapter 2: The Digital Drain... 49
Chapter 3: Redefining Success and Slowing Down................. 98
Chapter 4: Reconnecting With Your Body............................. 133
Chapter 5: Finding Mental Quiet in a Loud World 174
Chapter 6: Healing Relationships, Setting Boundaries......... 212
Chapter 7: Building Your Personal Calm Toolkit 247
Chapter 8: The Long Game — Living With Resilience and Hope 287
Conclusion: Your Calm is Not a Luxury — It's a Right 325
About the Author.. 332

Introduction

Welcome: You’re Not Alone

Let me start by saying this: if you're holding this book in your hands or reading it on a screen, chances are you’ve felt it too. That tightness in your chest that creeps in for no clear reason. The late-night overthinking that steals your sleep. The constant buzzing in your mind that refuses to quiet down even in your moments of rest.

You’re not broken. You’re not weak. You’re not alone.

In fact, you are part of what many experts are now calling the most anxious generation in history. And yet, strangely enough, nobody really talks about it in the way we need to hear it. Sure, you see social media posts, quick-fix reels, and a dozen wellness gurus telling you to meditate more or "just breathe," but let’s be honest: it rarely feels like enough.

What you need—what we all need—is not another list of to-dos or unrealistic ideals. What we need is to understand what’s happening, why it’s happening, and what we can actually do to feel human again.

That’s where this book comes in. And I want you to know that this isn’t some textbook filled with jargon or abstract theories. This is a conversation—between you and me. A friend talking to another friend. Real talk, real struggles, and real strategies.

So take a breath. Settle in. And let’s begin something honest together.

Why We're Talking About This

Anxiety isn't new. Humans have always felt fear, stress, and uncertainty. But something is different now, isn't it? Something about this moment in time has turned a manageable part of life into a permanent state of existence for so many of us.

We're always rushing. Always comparing. Always performing. And somewhere in all this noise, we've lost our calm.

We are more connected than ever, yet feel lonelier than ever. We have more information than any generation before us, but we're drowning in it. Our schedules are packed, our minds are overloaded, and our hearts are tired.

Whether you're a student navigating academic pressure, a parent juggling a thousand roles, an employee trying to stay relevant in a fast-changing world, or just someone trying to make sense of it all—anxiety has likely touched your life.

It shows up in small ways. Skipping meals. Mindless scrolling. Canceling plans. Overcommitting. Snapping at loved ones. Lying awake at night with racing thoughts. Or just feeling... off.

This book is about naming that feeling and exploring it without shame. Because when we understand it, we can begin to heal it.

What "Reclaiming Calm" Really Means

"Calm" doesn't mean you live on a mountain meditating for hours a day. It doesn't mean quitting your job and moving to a forest cabin. It doesn't even mean that you never feel stressed again.

Reclaiming calm means finding a steady, peaceful place within yourself that can exist even when the outside world is spinning. It means learning to breathe again—mentally, emotionally, spiritually. It means giving yourself permission to step off the hamster wheel of constant doing and start being.

It's about boundaries. About self-awareness. About paying attention to your inner world so that you can navigate the outer one with more grace.

Most importantly, reclaiming calm is not a luxury. It's your right. And you don't need anyone's permission to start reclaiming it today.

The Silent Epidemic: Living in Constant Anxiety

There was a time when anxiety was seen as a disorder, something unusual or clinical. Now, it feels like it's just part of the air we breathe.

People around the world are living in a quiet state of panic. Not always the loud, dramatic kind. Often it's subtle. Functional. Hidden behind a smile or disguised as ambition.

We've learned to normalize exhaustion. To joke about burnout. To glorify being busy as a badge of honor. But beneath that, many are suffering in silence.

Let's call it what it is: a silent epidemic.

This book isn't just for those diagnosed with anxiety. It's for anyone who has ever felt overwhelmed, emotionally tired, socially drained, mentally foggy, or spiritually disconnected.

Whether you live in bustling New York or a quiet town in India, whether you're in your early 20s figuring things out or in your 40s trying to keep things together, the emotional toll of modern life is a shared global experience.

How This Book Helps You — Practical, Friendly, and Real

Here's my promise to you: I'm not going to give you shallow advice or preach from a pedestal. This book is not about overnight fixes or becoming someone you're not.

Instead, I'll walk with you chapter by chapter through what anxiety really is, where it comes from, and how to navigate life with a sense of peace you thought you'd lost. You'll learn practical strategies—small, doable shifts that add up to meaningful change.

You'll also hear stories—some mine, some from others—that remind you you're not alone in how you feel. Because sometimes, just knowing that someone else understands is healing in itself.

This is a book you can read in bed after a long day. Or while sipping tea on a Sunday morning. Or even in the bathroom hiding from the chaos outside. Wherever you are, whenever you need it, let this book be a soft place to land.

Let's reclaim your calm together.

Let's begin.

Want Free Bonus Resources?
Take your calm journey deeper with these FREE, beautifully designed tools:

7-Day Calm Reset Challenge
Your Personal Calm Toolkit Printable
Anxious to Anchored: Daily Journal Template
The Anxious Generation Self-Test + Reflection Guide

Just send a quick email to: **EnochMerlyn@gmail.com**
with the subject **"Send My Calm Tools"** — and I'll personally email them to you!

Chapter 1: Understanding the Storm

Section 1: The Anxiety Generation — Why We're All On Edge

Imagine you wake up in the morning and before you even get out of bed, your phone buzzes. A message. A news alert. A reminder. A notification about someone's perfect life, someone's disaster, or something urgent you forgot to do yesterday. The moment your eyes open, you're already behind.

That's how many of us start our day. Not with a moment of silence, or a breath of gratitude, or even just stillness. We start with stress.

Welcome to the Anxiety Generation.

You might think you're the only one juggling a thousand thoughts at once, but the truth is, most people around you are doing the same—they're just not saying it out loud. And that silence? It has created a culture where we all feel like we have to keep pretending that we're okay.

But underneath the surface, we are fraying.

What's made our generation particularly prone to anxiety is not just biology or brain chemistry. It's culture. It's pace. It's the fact that we are living through massive shifts—economically, technologically, socially—without time to breathe or adjust.

Let's break this down.

**1. We're Always "On" ** You probably don't remember the last time you were truly disconnected. We carry our work, our social circles, our fears, our entertainment, and even our insecurities in our pockets.

Technology has given us amazing tools, but it has also blurred every boundary. You're checking work emails at dinner. You're watching world tragedies unfold in real time. You're trying to keep up with everyone, everywhere, all the time.

It's no wonder your nervous system feels hijacked.

2. The Pressure to Perform

There's an invisible scoreboard in modern life. Likes, follows, promotions, side hustles, highlight reels. It's exhausting. And it creates a constant fear of not measuring up.

Even if you don't care about social media, the pressure seeps in. You might compare your parenting to someone else's, your body to a fitness ad, your income to a friend's success story.

Comparison is no longer a thief of joy; it's a lifestyle.

3. Global Uncertainty

We're the generation raised on optimism, entering adulthood in chaos. Economic crashes, climate crises, pandemics, political divides. There is a low hum of dread in the background of our lives, and many of us don't even notice it anymore.

This global uncertainty shapes how we move through the world. We're afraid to plan too far ahead. We expect bad news. We're constantly bracing for impact.

4. Loss of Real-World Community

Ironically, we are more connected than ever but lonelier than ever. Virtual connection isn't the same as human connection.

We need touch. We need face-to-face laughter. We need someone to look into our eyes and say, "Me too." But the structures that once supported this—extended families, neighborhoods, community rituals—are fading.

5. The Myth of "Having It All"

Somewhere along the line, we were told we could have it all if we just worked hard enough. A thriving career. Perfect relationships. Sculpted bodies. Travel. Wealth. Influence.

What we weren't told is that trying to have it all at once can break us.

Life isn't meant to be a constant juggle of impossible expectations. And yet, when we inevitably fall short, we blame ourselves. We think we're failing when in fact, the system is broken.

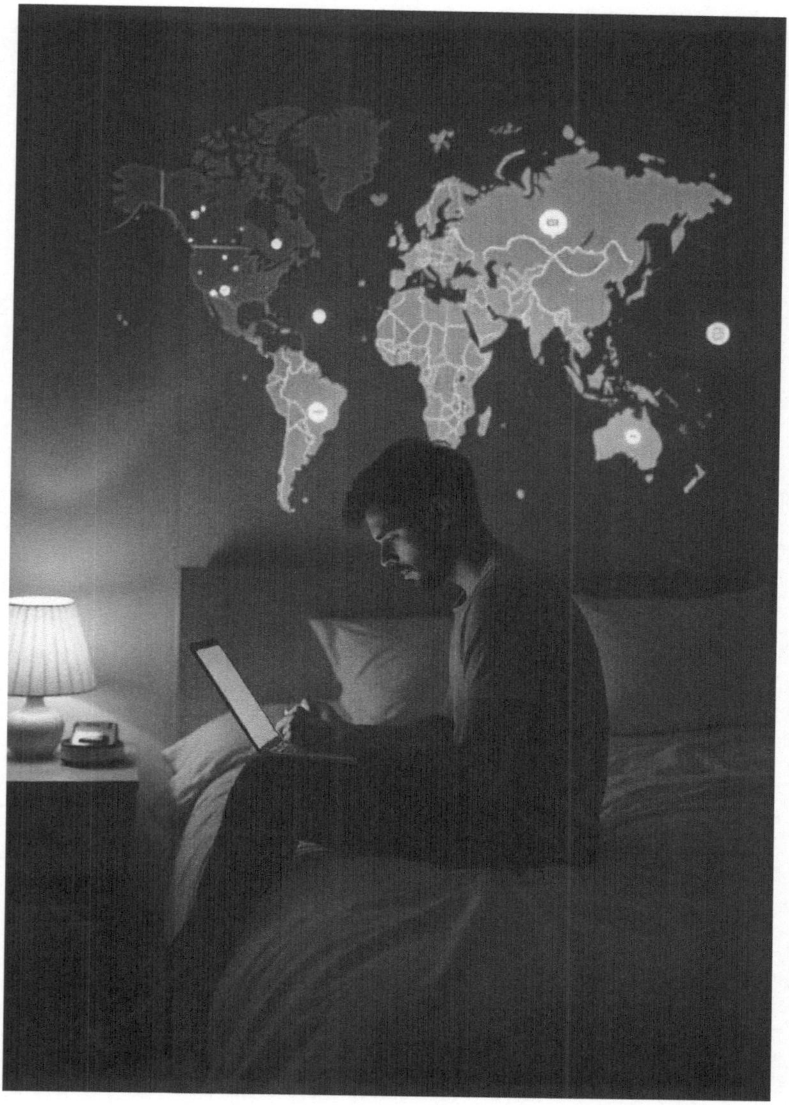

Closing Thought

Anxiety is not just a personal issue. It's a cultural signal. A message that something deeper needs our attention. And it starts with understanding why we feel the way we do.

The good news? Awareness is the first step. When you start to see the patterns, you can begin to untangle them. You can begin to breathe again.

Section 2: Breaking the Myth: It's Not Just in Your Head

Let's begin with a truth many of us need to hear: anxiety isn't just "in your head."

This phrase—often tossed around casually—is not only misleading, it's damaging. It reduces a complex, full-body experience to a mere thought problem, and that makes people feel like they're weak for not being able to "think" their way out of it.

But here's what you deserve to know: anxiety is not a flaw in your mindset. It is a whole-body, multi-system experience. It touches everything—your brain, your heart, your muscles, your digestion, your sleep, your relationships, and your sense of time and safety.

Understanding this is essential. Because once we stop blaming ourselves, we can start healing with compassion.

---

1. The Biology of Anxiety

Let's break down what actually happens when you feel anxious. Inside your brain is a little almond-shaped structure called the **amygdala**. It's your fear detector, and when it senses danger—real or imagined—it triggers your **fight, flight, or freeze** response.

Your brain sends signals to your body to prepare you for survival. Your heart starts racing. Your breathing gets shallow. Your muscles tense up. Your digestion slows down. Your pupils dilate.

It's a brilliant system—when you're facing an actual threat, like a wild animal.

But the problem is, in today's world, our threats look different. It could be a difficult email, a performance review, a crying child, or even an Instagram post that triggers comparison. Your brain still interprets them as threats. The body reacts the same way it would if you were running from danger.

In short: anxiety isn't "imagined." Your body is physically responding to emotional stress. It's real.

---

2. The Body Keeps the Score

This phrase, made famous by trauma researcher Bessel van der Kolk, perfectly captures the truth about anxiety. Your body remembers stress. And if you've been living in a state of chronic stress (which many people do), your body becomes conditioned to stay in that heightened state.

You may notice this as:

- Constant muscle tension (especially in your neck, jaw, or shoulders)

- Digestive issues (bloating, nausea, IBS)
- Racing heart or chest tightness
- Headaches or fatigue
- Difficulty falling asleep or staying asleep

These aren't random. They're your body's way of telling you something is off.

Your anxiety may not always show up as fear. Sometimes it shows up as irritability, perfectionism, forgetfulness, or physical illness. This is why simply "thinking positive" doesn't help much. Your body is already reacting—and it needs care, not criticism.

---

3. It's in Your Environment, Too

Anxiety isn't just internal—it's often reinforced by your environment.

Think about your daily life: constant notifications, background noise, multitasking, financial worries, social pressure. You might be living in a world that's overstimulating your nervous system every single day.

And if you grew up in an environment where emotions weren't acknowledged, or where survival meant staying alert, your brain may have learned to stay in a constant state of readiness. This "hypervigilance" doesn't go away overnight.

We must start seeing anxiety as a *normal reaction to abnormal demands*. It is not a personal failing. It is a message your body is sending about the weight it's carrying.

---

4. Cultural and Social Roots

Let's zoom out for a moment. Anxiety isn't experienced the same way across the world, but it does affect all of us. What differs is how it's understood and how it's treated.

In some cultures, talking about mental health is taboo. People suffer in silence because they fear judgment. In other places, anxiety is dismissed as laziness or lack of discipline.

The truth? Anxiety exists across all societies, ages, and backgrounds. What varies is whether it's named and addressed.

As a global community, we must start having honest conversations about emotional well-being. And that begins with understanding that anxiety is not weakness. It's a universal human response to an increasingly complex world.

---

5. The Role of Hormones and Nutrition

Let's talk briefly about two things we often overlook: **hormones and food.**

When your body is under chronic stress, it produces high levels of **cortisol**, the stress hormone. Over time, this can lead to fatigue, weight changes, sleep problems, and even anxiety loops. Hormonal changes during menstruation, postpartum, menopause, and thyroid issues can also make anxiety worse.

Then there's food. What you eat deeply affects how you feel. Processed food, excess sugar, and caffeine can disrupt your gut health—and your gut is home to about 90% of your **serotonin**, the "feel-good" neurotransmitter.

That means your stomach is talking to your brain, and it matters what you feed it.

We'll explore more on this in later chapters, but the bottom line is: your anxiety may have biological, environmental, and nutritional roots. That's why holistic approaches work best.

---

6. You Can't Heal What You Shame

When you believe that anxiety is just "in your head," you start to feel ashamed of it.

You might say things like:

- "What's wrong with me?"
- "Why can't I just get over this?"
- "Other people are dealing with worse."

But shame only deepens the wound. It tells you that your emotions are bad. That your needs are invalid. That your feelings are inconvenient.

Healing begins when you acknowledge your experience without judgment. When you treat your anxiety not as a flaw, but as a signal that something needs attention.

So let this be your permission slip: it's okay to feel this way. You're not making it up. You're not too sensitive. You are responding—wisely and instinctively—to an overwhelming world.

The goal isn't to "get rid" of anxiety completely. It's to understand it, work with it, and learn from it.

And that begins now.

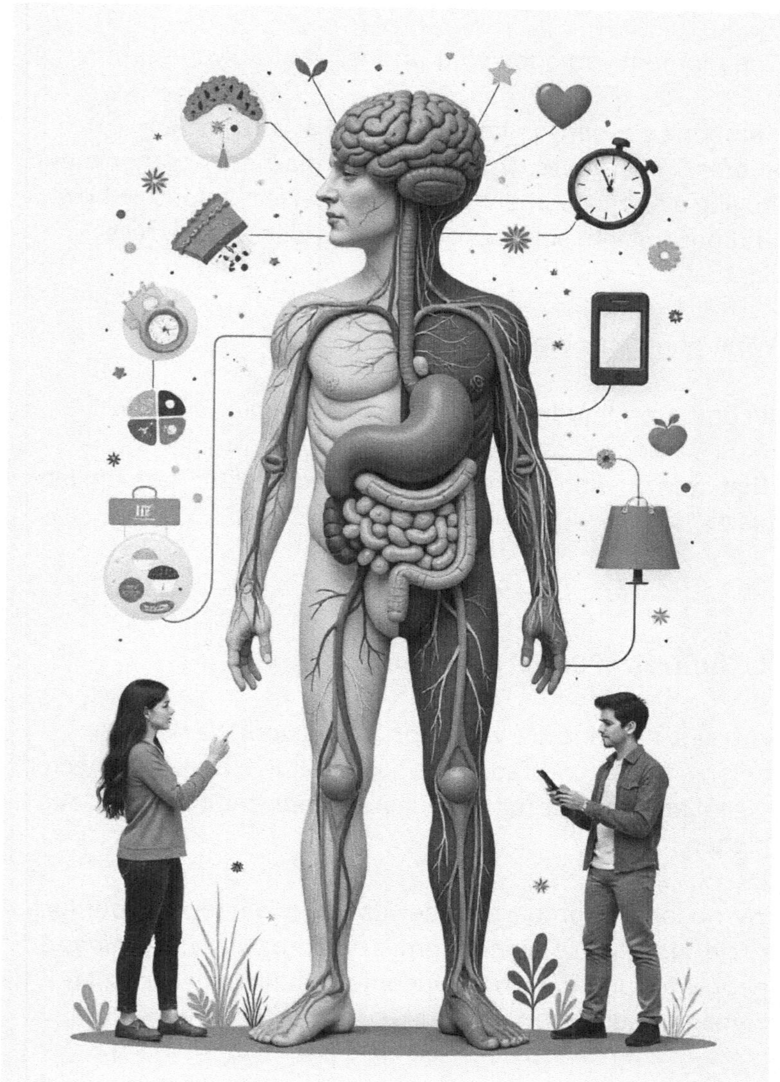

Section 3: Social Pressure, Hustle Culture, and Fear of Missing Out

Let's take a breath and look at the world we live in for a moment.

The moment you open your phone, what do you see?

Someone traveling in Italy. Someone else running a successful business. A friend getting married. Another friend buying a house. Someone making a perfect smoothie bowl and posting it at sunrise with glowing skin and perfect lighting.

What does your brain do?

It compares. It judges. It wonders, *"Am I doing enough?"*

That little question is where so much of our modern anxiety starts.

---

1. The Trap of Social Pressure

You see, humans are wired for connection. We want to belong, to be accepted, to be seen. But in a hyper-connected digital age, the bar for "belonging" keeps getting higher and higher.

We no longer compare ourselves to a few people in our local circle. Now, we're silently comparing ourselves to *millions* of people around the world—people with filters, editors, and highlight reels.

Social pressure isn't just about social media. It's in:

- The pressure to be constantly available
- The pressure to reply instantly
- The pressure to have an opinion on everything
- The pressure to achieve faster, bigger, louder

And it's exhausting.

When you're constantly trying to meet invisible standards, anxiety becomes inevitable.

---

2. Hustle Culture: The Myth That Productivity Equals Worth

Somewhere along the way, we began to believe that being "busy" means being valuable. That if we're not hustling, we're falling behind.

This idea has seeped into every corner of modern life:

- "Rise and grind."
- "Sleep when you're dead."
- "No days off."

Sounds motivating? Maybe at first. But long-term, it leads to burnout, not brilliance.

Let's be clear: working hard is not the enemy. But hustle culture glorifies *overwork*, often at the cost of health, relationships, and peace of mind. It praises those who sacrifice sleep and self-care in the name of achievement.

You start feeling guilty for resting. You feel behind if you take a day off. You wonder if you're wasting your potential simply because you didn't check off a 10-item to-do list before breakfast.

And all of this feeds anxiety. A chronic sense of, *"I'm not doing enough."*

But here's the truth: your worth is not tied to your output. You are not a machine. You are a human being, and you are allowed to exist without producing something every minute of the day.

---

3. The Fear of Missing Out (FOMO): The Anxiety of the Digital Age

FOMO is more than just a quirky acronym. It's a real emotional experience, and it's affecting millions of us without us even realizing it.

FOMO is the anxious feeling that something exciting, important, or fulfilling is happening somewhere else—and you're not part of it. It creates:

- Restlessness
- Dissatisfaction
- Impulsive decisions
- Difficulty being present

You might notice it when you scroll through photos of a party you weren't invited to. Or when your peers are making career moves and you're stuck in self-doubt. Or when you open Instagram and suddenly feel that your life is not enough.

FOMO convinces you that life is always better *elsewhere*. But it's a lie.

No one is living a perfect, unbroken string of joyful moments. What you're seeing is *curated*, not reality. And chasing other people's lives will only make you miss the beauty of your own.

---

4. The Algorithm Knows You're Anxious

Let's talk about tech for a moment.

Your phone doesn't just *show* you content—it *selects* it for you. Social media platforms use complex algorithms to keep you engaged by serving you posts that provoke strong emotions—fear, envy, outrage, and even anxiety.

Why? Because the longer you stay on the platform, the more ads they can show you.

That means:

- The more anxious you feel, the more you scroll.
- The more you compare, the more content you consume.
- The more you engage, the more your anxiety is fed.

The cycle repeats itself. And if we don't become aware of it, it starts to shape our entire worldview.

Awareness is your first line of defense. Recognize when your feed is feeding your fear.

---

5. Success Redefined: From External Validation to Inner Peace

It's time to ask an honest question:

What does success mean to you—really?

If success only means looking good to others, being busy, being admired, or constantly winning, then you will always be anxious. Because these things depend on *external* validation.

True success feels different. It's quiet. It feels like:

- Doing work you care about
- Being kind to yourself
- Having time for rest
- Being present with loved ones
- Feeling safe in your body

We're allowed to want ambition and achievement. But when it comes from a place of fear or insecurity, it leads to burnout. When it comes from self-respect and clarity, it becomes sustainable.

Reclaiming calm means letting go of what you *should* be doing, and listening more closely to what your heart *needs*.

---

6. Reclaiming Presence in a Noisy World

In a world that's always telling you to move faster, think more, be more—**presence** is revolutionary.

Presence means you are here, now. You are not in the past, not stuck in "what ifs," and not racing toward the next achievement. You are breathing. You are noticing. You are living.

This is one of the most powerful tools against anxiety. Because presence is where peace lives.

But presence takes practice. It takes:

- Slowing down
- Turning off notifications
- Creating screen boundaries
- Having honest conversations
- Journaling, breathing, walking, noticing

When we reclaim presence, we reclaim power. We shift our attention from the artificial noise of comparison to the real life unfolding around us.

And slowly, the anxious storm begins to calm.

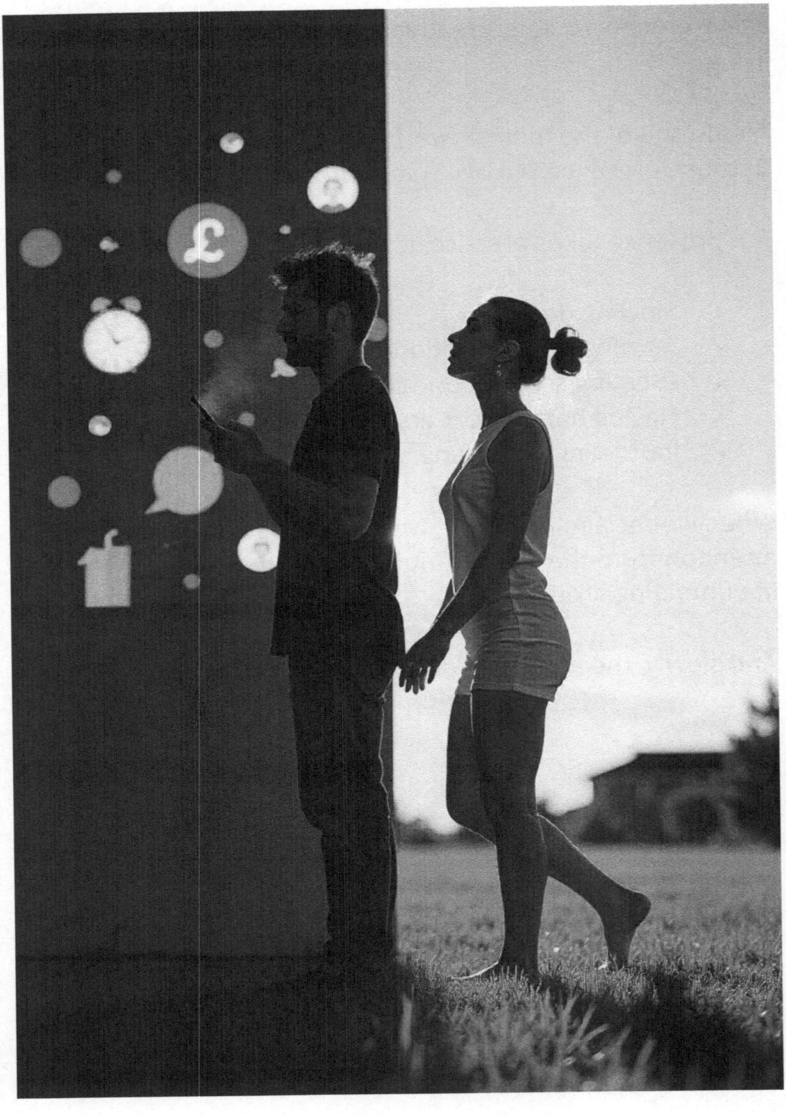

Section 4: The Cost of Always Being "On"

Let's talk about something most of us don't even realize we're doing: living life in "always-on" mode.

You wake up and immediately check your phone. You reply to messages while brushing your teeth. You skim emails over breakfast. You answer work calls on your commute. You scroll through notifications at dinner. You go to bed... still wired.

It's like our brains never get to power down.

In today's world, we're constantly connected, constantly engaged, constantly *on*. And while this might seem productive—or even normal—it comes at a cost. A big one.

---

1. The Hidden Energy Drain

Being mentally "on" all the time isn't just tiring—it's *draining*. Every alert, every ping, every decision, every swipe—it all adds up.

Our brains weren't designed for this kind of nonstop stimulation. The human nervous system evolved for cycles of activity and rest, focus and pause. But the modern world has flattened those cycles into one long, never-ending push.

And when your brain doesn't get a break?

- You feel foggy.
- You struggle to concentrate.
- You're more irritable.
- You sleep poorly.

- You start feeling anxious... and you don't even know why.

It's like your internal battery never gets the chance to recharge.

---

2. The Myth of Multitasking

Let's bust a popular myth: *Multitasking does not make you more efficient.*

In fact, research shows it actually makes you less productive and more stressed.

When you switch from one task to another—say, checking a notification while writing an email—your brain goes through what's called "cognitive switching." This creates a lag. A tiny moment of readjustment. Now multiply that by hundreds of switches a day.

The result?

- You feel scattered.
- You make more mistakes.
- You finish tasks slower.
- Your anxiety quietly increases.

It's like your brain is trying to juggle too many balls—and some always drop.

---

3. The Rise of Hypervigilance

"Always being on" doesn't just affect your mind. It also affects your *body*.

You might not realize it, but many people today live in a state of low-grade fight-or-flight mode. It's called **hypervigilance**—when your nervous system is constantly scanning for threats, stressors, or incoming demands.

Even if you don't feel "panicked," your body might be holding:

- Tension in your shoulders
- Shallow breathing
- A racing heart
- Tightness in your stomach

These are signs that your nervous system is overloaded. And the more it happens, the more anxious you feel—without even knowing why.

Your body is saying, "I need a break." But we often push through until burnout hits.

---

4. The Erosion of Boundaries

One of the biggest culprits of anxiety today is the collapse of boundaries.

Work follows us home. Messages come at all hours. Social media never sleeps.

Once upon a time, there were natural boundaries: clocks, commutes, weekends, phone-free dinners. But now, those lines are blurry at best.

The result is what experts call "boundary fatigue"—where we no longer know when to stop, rest, or say no.

Without boundaries:

- Work bleeds into family time
- Social updates interrupt real conversations
- Your brain never fully enters "rest mode"

And this chronic blur makes anxiety feel like your new normal.

---

5. The Sleep Crisis

Let's not overlook the quiet casualty of being always "on": *sleep*.

Many people today are experiencing sleep issues—not because they don't want to sleep, but because their brains won't slow down. Being constantly stimulated through screens, notifications, noise, and overthinking takes a toll.

Poor sleep leads to:

- Weakened immunity
- Reduced focus and memory
- Increased emotional reactivity
- Amplified anxiety symptoms

It becomes a vicious cycle: anxiety disrupts sleep, and poor sleep increases anxiety.

Your mind needs *off-time* to process, reset, and heal. And sleep is one of the most powerful ways your body does that.

---

6. What Happens When We Never Pause

If you were to drive your car non-stop, refill the fuel but never service it, never turn off the engine, never let it rest—what would happen?

It would break down.

The same is true for us. When we're always on, we start to lose:

- Our sense of joy
- Our creativity
- Our patience
- Our ability to connect

Eventually, our mental health begins to fray. Not because we're weak—but because we're human.

We're not meant to be alert 24/7. We're meant to ebb and flow, to engage and disengage, to work and to rest.

The good news? We can choose to step off the hamster wheel. We can reclaim our time, our peace, and our calm.

Reclaiming the "Off" Button

The antidote to always being on is *intentional off-time*.

This doesn't mean quitting your job or going off the grid. It means building small, sacred spaces in your day where your mind can breathe.

Try this:

- **Tech boundaries:** Set a "digital sunset" time each night where you unplug from devices.
- **Focus windows:** Work in short, focused bursts with intentional breaks.
- **Mindful transitions:** Pause for 1 minute between tasks to reset your nervous system.
- **Screen-free mornings:** Give your brain 30 minutes of quiet before diving into the digital world.

These moments of pause aren't luxuries—they're necessities.

When we rest, we heal. When we unplug, we reset. When we pause, we gain clarity.

This is how we begin to reclaim calm in a noisy world.

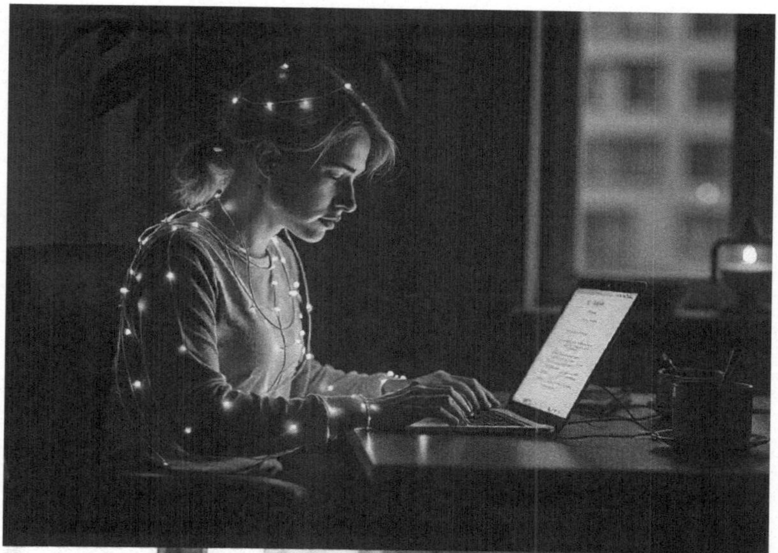

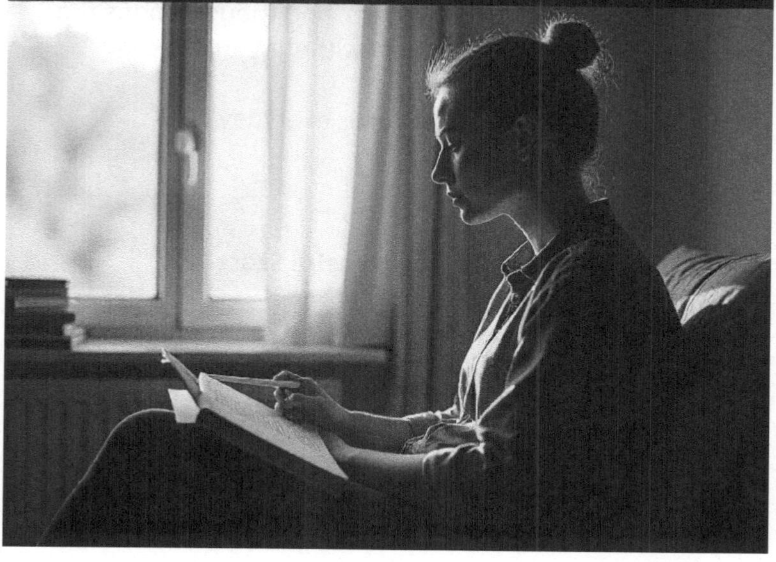

Section 5: Recognizing the Patterns in Your Own Life

Before we can change anything, we have to *see* it.

It's one thing to talk about anxiety, hustle culture, and the cost of being always "on." It's another thing entirely to realize how these things show up in *your* daily life. We often think we're fine—just tired, a little overworked, maybe a bit distracted. But beneath those everyday feelings, there might be deeper patterns quietly fueling our anxiety.

Recognizing these patterns isn't about blaming yourself. It's about becoming aware, with curiosity and kindness.

This chapter is your mirror. We're going to walk through how to spot the small behaviors, habits, and thought loops that contribute to your anxiety, often without you noticing.

Let's explore the landscape of your everyday life.

---

1. Your Morning Routine: A Stressful Start?

How you start your day sets the tone for everything that follows. Many people begin their mornings in reactive mode—scrolling their phones, replying to emails, rushing through routines.

Ask yourself:

- Do you check your phone within 5 minutes of waking up?
- Do you feel behind before you even get out of bed?
- Is your mind already racing with to-do lists?

These moments matter. A stressful morning creates a low-level hum of urgency that can stay with you all day.

Try This: Track your first 30 minutes after waking up. What do you do? How do you feel? Where can you build in 5 minutes of calm?

---

2. Decision Fatigue Throughout the Day

Every day, we make hundreds—sometimes thousands—of decisions. From what to wear to how to respond to a message, each choice pulls a little bit of energy from your mental reserves.

Decision fatigue doesn't just make us tired. It can make us anxious. When we're overloaded with choices, our brains start to panic.

Patterns to Watch For:

- Indecisiveness over small things
- Mental exhaustion by late afternoon
- Feeling overwhelmed when plans change

Recognizing these signs helps you plan your day with fewer mental drains.

Try This: Create mini-rituals: a default breakfast, a go-to outfit, a simple "wind-down" routine. Fewer decisions = more calm.

---

3. The Hidden Language of Self-Talk

We all have an inner voice. Sometimes it's kind and encouraging. Other times... not so much.

The way you talk to yourself *matters*. It shapes your emotional state, your confidence, and your anxiety levels.

Start Noticing:

- Do you talk to yourself like a critic or a coach?
- What phrases do you repeat when you're stressed?
- Would you speak to a friend the way you speak to yourself?

Negative self-talk isn't just background noise—it creates tension in your body and unease in your mind.

Try This: Whenever you catch a critical thought, ask: *Is this true? Is this kind? Is this helpful?*

---

4. Emotional Checkpoints: Where Does Stress Build Up?

Your body is always communicating. Tension, tightness, and racing thoughts are signals—not just symptoms.

Throughout your day, certain moments might repeatedly spark anxiety:

- Opening your inbox
- Receiving a Slack message
- Walking into a meeting
- Picking up your child from school

We call these *emotional checkpoints*. They're worth noticing.

Map Your Stress: Keep a journal for one day. Every time you feel stressed, pause and write what happened, how you felt, and what you were doing. You might start to see a pattern.

Over time, these patterns can help you make smarter adjustments.

---

5. The Role of Environment

Your environment subtly influences your mental state. It can either calm or agitate you. Cluttered spaces, loud noises, constant background screens—all these can create micro-stressors.

Ask yourself:

- Do you feel more anxious in certain rooms?
- Does your workspace feel chaotic or peaceful?
- Is your phone always in your line of sight?

Small environmental changes can lead to big emotional shifts.

Try This: Designate a "calm corner" in your home—one screen-free space for quiet reflection, reading, or just breathing.

---

6. Your Relationship with Time

Time anxiety is real. It's the feeling of never having enough. It's being haunted by the clock. It's the guilt of resting when there's more to do.

Do these sound familiar?

- "I should've done more today."
- "I'll relax once I finish this."
- "Why does the weekend go by so fast?"

Many of us have an unhealthy relationship with time—and it shows up as anxiety.

Shift Your Language: Instead of saying *I don't have time*, try *It's not a priority right now.* It brings clarity—and puts you back in control.

---

7. The Loop of Overcommitment

Do you say yes when you mean no? Do you take on more than you can handle? Do you fill every available slot in your schedule?

This pattern is deeply connected to anxiety. We overcommit out of fear—of missing out, of disappointing others, of seeming lazy.

Watch for These Signals:

- Dreading your calendar
- Resenting plans you agreed to

- Canceling at the last minute because you're overwhelmed

Learning to honor your limits is one of the most powerful steps toward reclaiming calm.

Try This: Every time someone asks for your time, pause and ask yourself: *Will this drain me or energize me?*

Why Noticing Patterns Matters

You can't change what you don't recognize.

When you begin to see these patterns—not with judgment, but with curiosity—you gain insight. And with insight comes power.

It's not about being perfect. It's about *being aware*. Awareness gives you the freedom to choose something different.

Remember: calm isn't something you wait for. It's something you *create*—moment by moment, choice by choice.

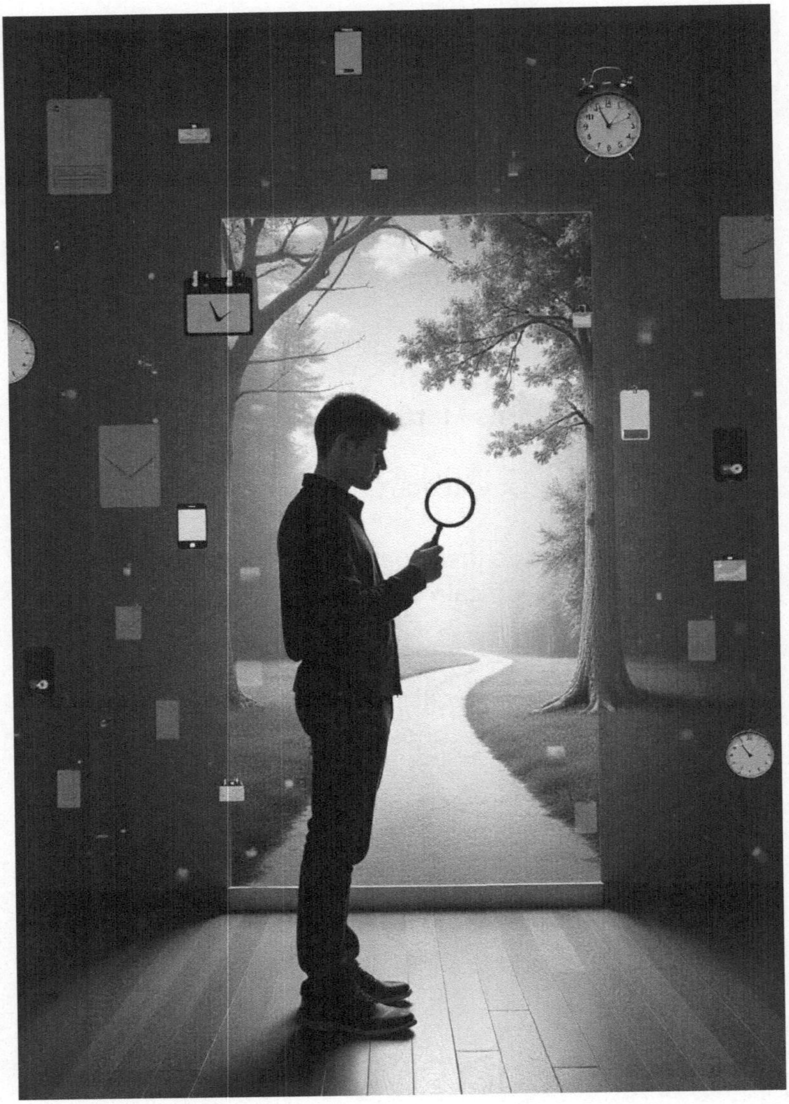

Section 6: First Step Toward Calm — Self-Awareness Without Shame

So, you've begun to see it—the patterns, the pressures, the background buzz of anxiety you've maybe lived with so long it feels normal. That awareness? It's powerful. It's your first real step toward calm.

But here's the key: You must take this step without shame.

If there's one thing we need to clear up right now, it's this—*there's nothing wrong with you.*

You are not broken. You're not weak. You're not "too sensitive."

You are a human being, living in a very overwhelming world.

And the fact that you're reading this, noticing your patterns, and wanting to reclaim your peace? That speaks to your strength.

Let's talk about how to walk forward—gently, honestly, and without judgment.

---

1. Awareness Is Not Blame

Sometimes, when we finally see something clearly—like how we've been saying yes to everyone but ourselves, or how our phones have become pacifiers—we feel a wave of guilt or embarrassment.

Don't.

Awareness is not about self-blame. It's about *self-honoring*.

Imagine looking at your life like a map. You're not mad at the map for showing you where you are. You're just using it to find where to go next.

You can love yourself and still want to grow. You can accept yourself and still want to change. These are not opposites—they're partners.

---

2. The Gentle Power of Naming

One of the simplest, most effective tools for reducing anxiety is naming what's happening.

Noticing and saying, "I'm overwhelmed because I haven't had quiet all day." Or, "I'm feeling tension because I've had 10 notifications in the last hour."

Naming helps you:

- Ground your experience in reality.
- Reduce emotional swirl.
- Interrupt automatic responses.

You shift from being *in* the storm to *observing* the storm. That's where calm begins.

Try This: Whenever you feel anxious, pause and describe what's happening like a weather report: "It feels cloudy right now. There's a storm of expectation moving in. I need shelter."

---

3. The Shame Spiral — and How to Step Out of It

Shame is a sneaky emotion. It doesn't just say "I made a mistake." It says, "I *am* a mistake."

When we're dealing with anxiety, shame often rides shotgun:

- You feel anxious → You avoid tasks.
- You avoid tasks → You feel guilty.
- You feel guilty → You criticize yourself.
- You criticize yourself → You feel more anxious.

This cycle can feel endless.

The Exit Ramp: Self-compassion.

Every time you speak kindly to yourself, you break the spiral.

Say it with me:

"I'm doing the best I can with what I have. And that is enough for today."

This is not a cheesy affirmation. This is a *lifeline*.

---

4. Curiosity Over Criticism

A curious mind is an open mind. A critical mind is a closed one.

Instead of saying, "Why am I like this?" try, "Isn't it interesting that I always feel anxious before opening my email?"

Curiosity leads to:

- Gentle self-exploration
- Playful problem-solving
- Emotional openness

Criticism leads to:

- Emotional shutdown
- Harsh self-judgment
- Defensiveness

Start treating yourself like a scientist studying a beloved subject—not a judge passing a sentence.

Try This: Keep a "curiosity journal." At the end of each day, ask: "What did I learn about myself today?"

---

5. Calm Isn't a Destination — It's a Daily Choice

If you're waiting for a perfect moment when everything is done, everyone is happy, and the world is quiet... you'll be waiting a long time.

Calm isn't some magical place you arrive at one day. It's something you *practice*.

Every deep breath. Every boundary you set. Every moment you pause to check in with yourself. These are the building blocks of peace.

And some days, it won't be easy. But over time, it becomes easier. Like muscle memory. Like riding a bike.

You don't need to *become* a calm person. You already *are*. You just need to clear the noise to meet yourself again.

6. Permission to Go Slow

We're conditioned to want fast fixes. "Give me 5 hacks to stop feeling anxious."

But the truth is—lasting change takes time.

You have permission to go slow. To take this one step at a time. To repeat lessons. To stumble. To circle back.

Healing is not a straight line. It's a spiral staircase.

And even on the days you feel like you've gone backwards, you're still moving. Still growing. Still showing up.

That's enough. *You're enough.*

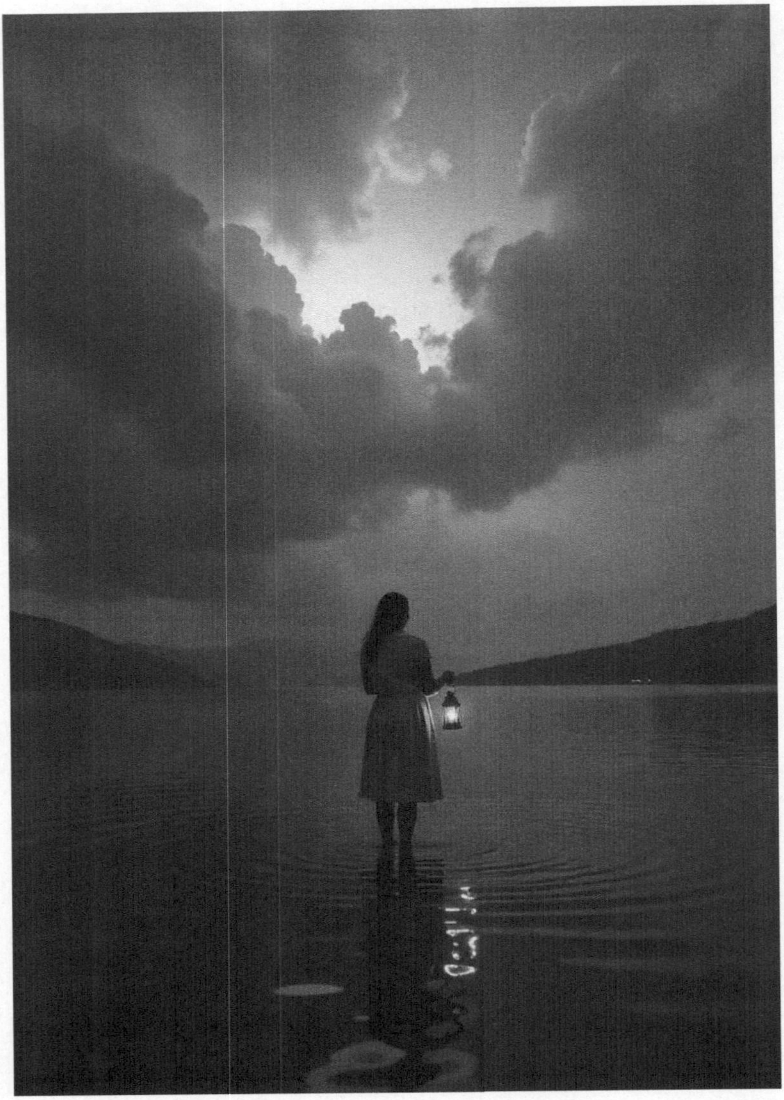

Chapter 1 Summary: Understanding the Storm

We began this journey by calling out a truth many feel but few say aloud—anxiety has become our baseline. From the unrelenting pace of modern life to the subtle (and not-so-subtle) social pressures, from digital noise to the weight of constant expectations, many of us are simply exhausted.

In Section 1, we explored how this generation has come to wear anxiety like a second skin, and why it's not your fault.

In Section 2, we debunked the myth that anxiety is all "in your head," recognizing its very real impact on our bodies, thoughts, and behavior.

In Section 3, we uncovered how hustle culture, social media, and fear of missing out have become silent contributors to chronic overwhelm.

In Section 4, we looked at the toll of always being "on"—mentally, emotionally, and physically.

Section 5 invited you to recognize your personal anxiety patterns—those daily micro-stressors that sneak into your routine unnoticed.

And in this final section, we affirmed that awareness is your first, most powerful tool—and that you don't need to carry shame for feeling how you feel.

The storm is real. But so is your strength. And now, with clarity and compassion, you've taken the most important step:

You've *seen* it.

You've *named* it.

And together, we're learning how to *navigate* it.

In the chapters to come, we'll explore practical strategies to shift out of survival mode and into a life that feels calmer, more grounded, and more joyfully human.

You're not alone. You're not behind. You're right on time.

Let's keep going.

Chapter 2: The Digital Drain

Section 1: Scrolling and Stress — The Hidden Connection

You wake up, roll over, and reach for your phone before you've even said good morning to the day. Notifications. Updates. Alerts. It begins — the endless scroll.

What started as a quick check turns into 20 minutes. Before your feet even touch the ground, your brain is already buzzing. And you tell yourself it's just part of modern life.

But here's a truth many of us are only beginning to admit:

Our screens are stealing our calm.

Let's talk about why.

---

1. The Promise vs. The Reality of Connection

We live in a world where we are more connected than ever — at least digitally. We can text across continents, video call from different time zones, and share our lives in a few taps.

The promise? Instant connection. The reality? Constant stimulation.

We aren't just connected to people anymore. We're connected to *feeds*. To *noise*. To *comparison*.

You might go to check on a friend and end up feeling bad about your own life. You might open your phone for peace and end up with panic.

Social media, messaging apps, news updates — they all keep you plugged in. But being constantly plugged in drains your battery more than you realize.

---

2. Doomscrolling and Anxiety: What the Brain Feels

Let's get into what really happens when you scroll — especially through bad news, controversy, or overly curated highlight reels.

Your brain processes this information like it's happening to *you*. Your nervous system doesn't know the difference between a real threat and a digital one.

Every time you read upsetting news, your body activates a mild stress response. Every time you see someone's perfect life, your brain compares. Every swipe is a tiny jolt.

Now multiply that by hundreds — even thousands — per day. No wonder we're fried.

Psychologists have coined the term "doomscrolling" to describe the act of endlessly consuming negative content. It keeps us in a loop of:

- Anxiety
- Numbness
- Restlessness

And we call that 'relaxing time.'

---

3. Micro-Stress, Macro-Impact

Not every notification feels like a crisis. But together, they stack up.

Each buzz, ping, or red dot triggers a micro-stress response:

- Increased heart rate
- Spike in cortisol
- Disrupted focus

Over time, these micro-stresses can:

- Disrupt sleep patterns
- Increase irritability
- Weaken attention span
- Contribute to burnout

We underestimate the impact because it feels so small. But it's like being pricked by a pin a hundred times a day — it adds up.

---

4. The Attention Tug-of-War

Have you ever noticed how hard it is to finish a book or sit through a movie these days?

It's not just you.

Smartphones train your brain to crave fast rewards. Every like, every scroll, every quick hit of novelty — it's a dopamine trickle.

Your mind learns:

"Why sit in silence when you can scroll?" "Why focus deeply when you can be distracted instantly?"

We are losing the ability to just *be*. To *pause*. To *breathe*.

This loss of attention isn't just inconvenient. It fuels anxiety, because your brain is constantly switching gears without rest.

---

5. Comparison Culture and Self-Worth

Let's talk about one of the quietest, most corrosive parts of the digital drain: comparison.

We don't just scroll for entertainment — we scroll for identity.

And often, what we see are:

- Perfect photos
- Highlight reels
- Filtered joy

Rarely do we see:

- The messy middle
- The bad days
- The anxious moments

But we compare our *reality* to someone else's *presentation*. And we lose.

This fuels a subtle form of anxiety — the belief that you're behind, not enough, or missing out.

And the worst part? We do it over and over again, without even noticing.

---

6. Sleep and the Blue Light Cycle

How many nights have you told yourself, "Just five more minutes," only to find it's midnight and you're still on your phone?

Screens disrupt sleep in two big ways:

1. **Blue light:** It tells your brain it's still daytime, delaying melatonin production.
2. **Mental stimulation:** News, messages, reels — they keep your mind alert when it should be winding down.

Poor sleep leads to poor emotional regulation. Poor regulation leads to more stress. And more stress leads to more late-night scrolling. It's a loop.

Try This:

- Set a digital curfew (no screens 30 minutes before bed).
- Charge your phone outside the bedroom.
- Use a warm-tone screen filter in the evening.

7. Replacing Scrolling with Stillness

The solution isn't throwing your phone in the ocean. It's learning to reclaim your *agency*.

Start noticing:

- When do you reach for your phone?
- What are you avoiding when you scroll?
- How do you feel *after*?

Then experiment with replacing 5 minutes of scrolling with:

- Breathing deeply
- Journaling your thoughts
- Taking a short walk
- Doing absolutely nothing

Stillness is a skill. And you can build it.

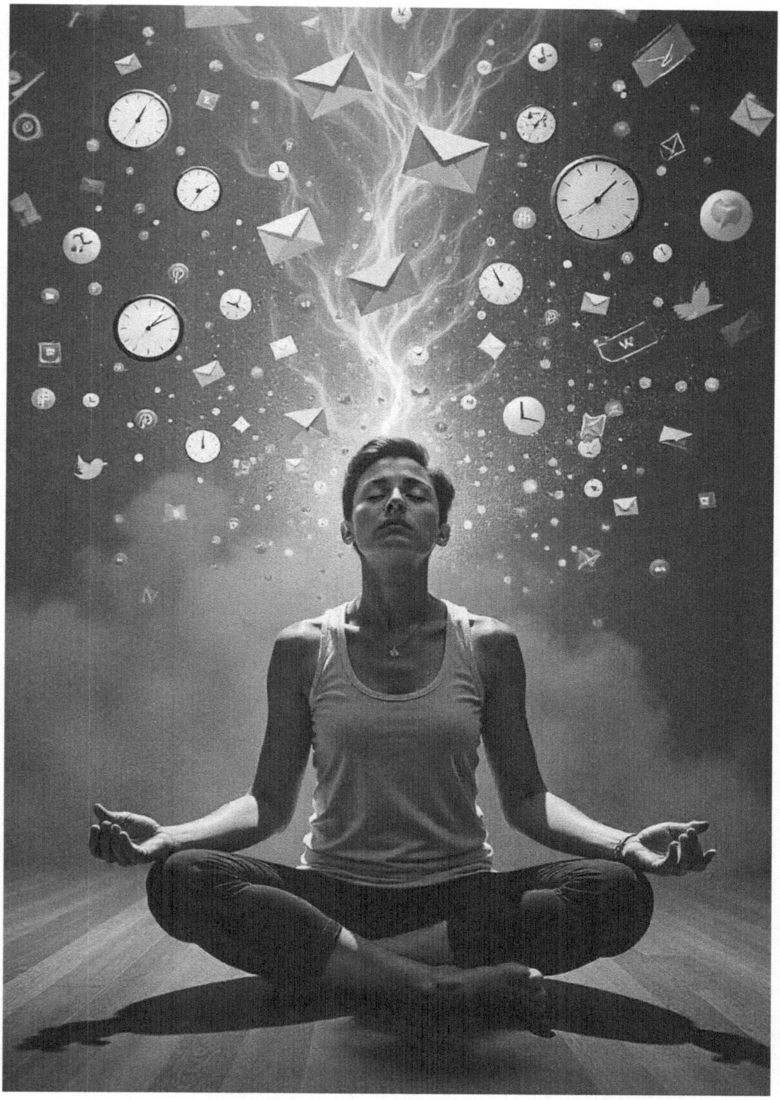

Section 2: Doomscrolling, Notifications, and the Rise of "Techxiety"

Imagine this: You're trying to relax after a long day. You sit down with a warm drink, maybe even light a candle. You exhale. Finally, a moment of peace.

Then—*ping.*

Your hand reaches for your phone almost without thinking. One message becomes two. A news alert. A social media update. The candle's flickering glow fades into the background. You're back in the whirlpool again.

And you didn't even mean to be.

That's the story of **techxiety** — a new kind of stress born from our digital age.

---

1. What Is "Techxiety" Anyway?

"Techxiety" is a term coined to describe the persistent, low-grade anxiety that stems from our relationship with technology. It's not in your head — it's in your *habits*.

Techxiety is:

- That twitch you feel to check your phone every few minutes.
- The unease that rises when you're without Wi-Fi.
- The restlessness after too much screen time.
- The pressure to always respond, always stay updated, always be reachable.

It's our nervous system slowly fraying under the weight of constant digital stimulation.

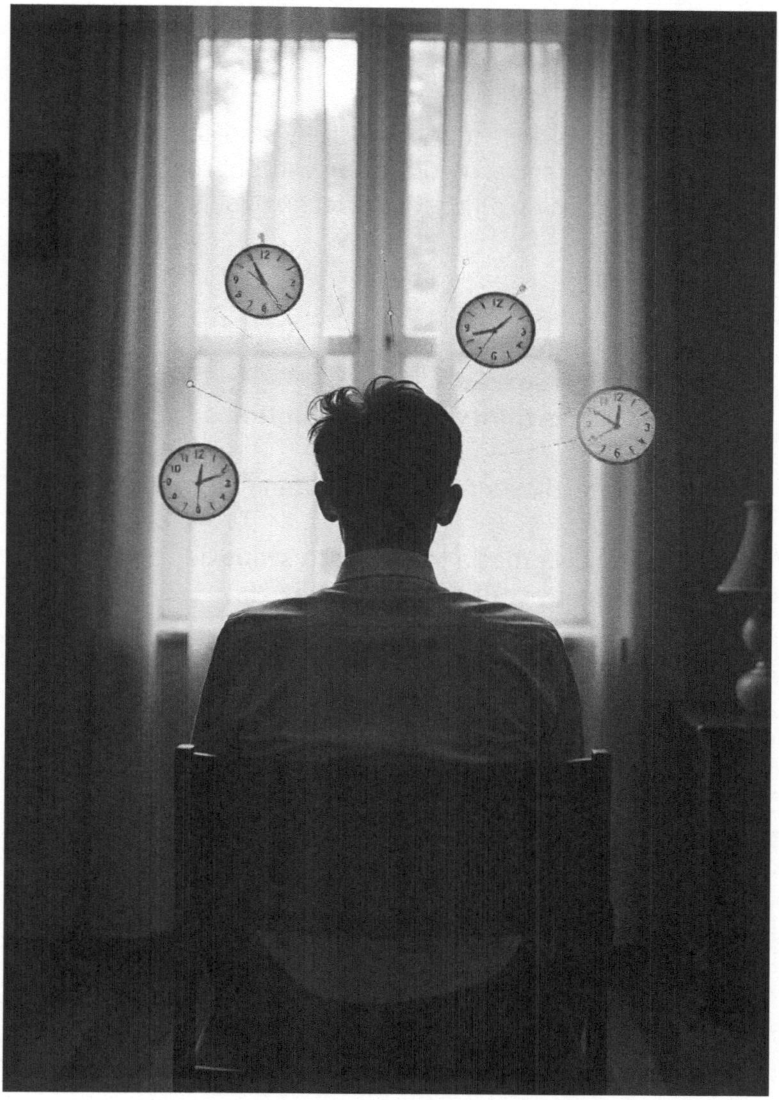

2. Doomscrolling: The Addiction to Bad News

We touched on doomscrolling earlier, but let's dive deeper here — because it's one of the most powerful drivers of techxiety.

Doomscrolling is the act of obsessively scrolling through negative news or social media, often without realizing how much time is passing or how it's affecting you.

Why do we do it?

- **To feel informed.**
- **To feel prepared.**
- **To find certainty in uncertain times.**

But instead of feeling informed, we often feel overwhelmed.

Each headline becomes a threat. Each swipe adds weight. Each update keeps your brain on edge.

Even worse, doomscrolling is designed to be endless. Social media platforms and news apps are built to keep you engaged — using algorithms that serve up fear, controversy, and emotional triggers. Why? Because it keeps you scrolling.

---

3. The Neurological Toll

Let's get into the brain science.

When you receive a notification or read dramatic news:

- Your **amygdala** (the brain's fear center) is activated.

- Your **sympathetic nervous system** gears up for "fight or flight."
- Your **dopamine system** is tickled — giving you tiny hits of pleasure that keep you coming back.

The result? A brain stuck in a loop of craving and stress.

And this loop doesn't just affect your emotional state. It also disrupts:

- Sleep quality
- Short-term memory
- Ability to focus
- Emotional regulation

In short, techxiety doesn't just feel uncomfortable — it *changes* how your brain functions.

---

4. Notifications: A Constant Call to Attention

Let's pause and count: How many apps send you notifications daily?

Now multiply that by the number of times you pick up your phone to check them.

The average person gets over **60–100 notifications per day** — and that's on the low end.

Each ping or buzz demands your attention. And even if you don't respond, your brain still registers it. That tiny moment of "What was that?" is a form of mental tension.

In psychology, this is called **intermittent reinforcement** — the same principle used in slot machines. You never know when the next reward (message, like, update) will appear, so your brain stays in a heightened state of anticipation.

It's exhausting.

And it's *normalized*.

---

5. The Myth of Multitasking

Notifications are one part of the story. The other part is how they fragment our attention.

You might think you're multitasking when you:

- Reply to emails while listening to a podcast.
- Scroll Instagram while watching Netflix.
- Answer texts during work meetings.

But neuroscience tells us: **Multitasking is a myth.**

What we're really doing is **task-switching** — rapidly jumping between focuses. And this:

- Increases mental fatigue
- Reduces productivity
- Raises stress levels

The human brain isn't wired for constant context shifts. Every ding is a derailment.

Over time, this disconnection from *deep focus* leads to a more shallow, distracted way of living — and yes, more techxiety.

6. "Always On" Culture and Its Psychological Cost

Whether it's your boss expecting instant replies or your group chat lighting up at 1 a.m., we're living in an "always-on" culture.

This constant availability:

- Blurs the line between work and rest.
- Replaces quiet moments with stimulation.
- Turns silence into something we fear, not seek.

What's lost in this digital barrage is *presence*. Real, grounded, slow presence — the kind where your nervous system resets, your thoughts settle, and your heart rate slows.

When we lose that, anxiety becomes a baseline.

---

7. What You Can Do — Without Tossing Your Phone

You don't have to disappear into a forest or throw your phone into the sea to heal from techxiety.

Here are practical ways to start reclaiming your digital calm:

1. Audit your notifications

- Turn off non-essential alerts.
- Set "Do Not Disturb" windows.

2. Introduce tech boundaries

- No phones during meals.
- Phone-free zones (like the bedroom).

3. Schedule scrolling

- Give yourself dedicated scroll time.
- Stick to it.

4. Replace digital noise with analog calm

- Read a paper book.
- Go for a walk.
- Journal with a pen.

5. Use "tech check-ins" Ask yourself:

- Why am I picking up my phone right now?
- What am I hoping to feel?
- What do I feel after I use it?

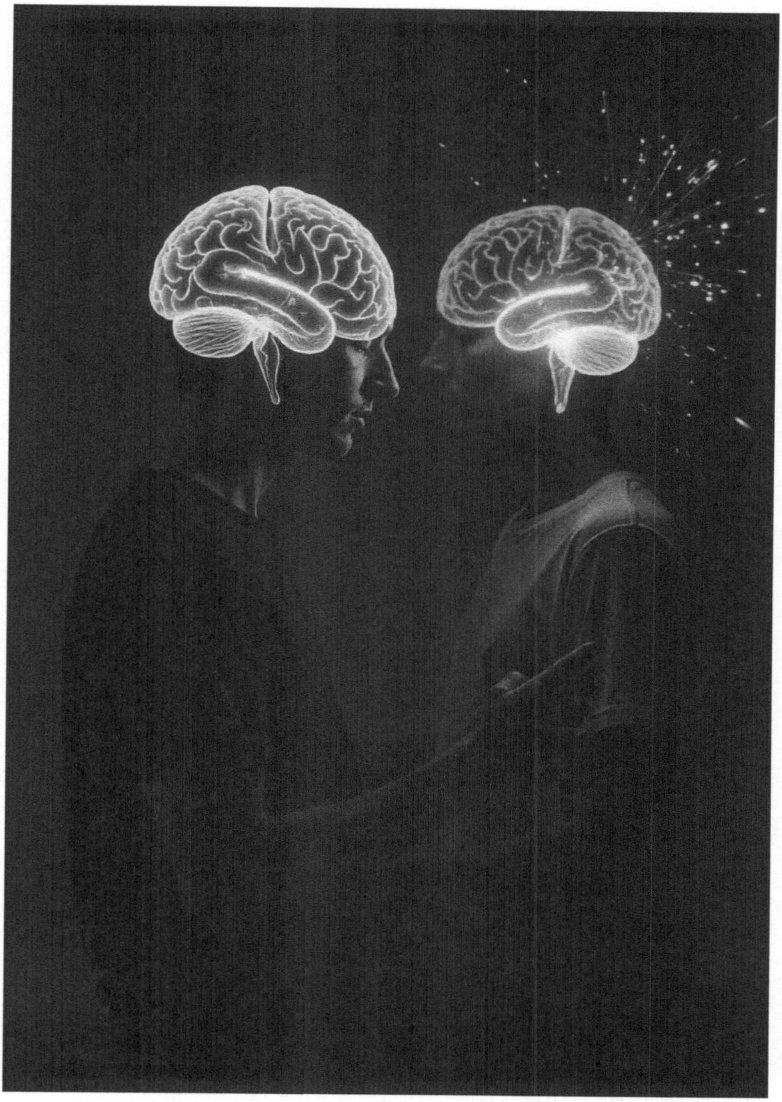

Section 3: How Comparison Culture Eats at Our Peace

Let's be honest. Most of us don't scroll through social media for information — we scroll to *feel something.*

Sometimes we want connection. Sometimes we want to escape. But often, without realizing it, we're scrolling to see where we stand in the invisible race that plays out on our screens every day.

And that's where comparison begins.

---

1. The Illusion of "Everyone Else"

Social media was supposed to connect us. Instead, it's made us spectators of each other's highlight reels.

You open Instagram or TikTok and what do you see?

- Friends posting vacation selfies in exotic locations.
- Entrepreneurs sharing their six-figure success stories.
- Parents displaying picture-perfect family dinners.
- Fitness influencers flaunting their "just woke up like this" bodies.

It looks like *everyone else* has it figured out — while you're still trying to get through your day without burning out.

But here's the truth: What you're seeing isn't reality. It's *curated* content.

No one posts their:

- Financial stress

- Marriage struggles
- Messy kitchens
- Mental health relapses

So you're comparing your behind-the-scenes to someone else's carefully edited front stage. And the result? Anxiety, inadequacy, and a quiet erosion of peace.

---

2. The Psychology of Comparison

Psychologists call it **social comparison theory** — the idea that we determine our own social and personal worth based on how we stack up against others.

There are two types:

- **Upward comparison:** Comparing yourself to someone you think is "better off."
- **Downward comparison:** Comparing yourself to someone you think is "worse off."

While downward comparison can briefly boost your ego, *upward comparison* is more common — and more dangerous.

Why? Because it often leads to:

- **Imposter syndrome** ("I'll never be as good as them.")
- **Envy and resentment**
- **Perfectionism**
- **Depression and burnout**

And here's the kicker — the person you're comparing yourself to might be doing the exact same thing, looking at *someone else.*

It's a loop that has no finish line.

---

3. Metrics and Mental Health

Social media has gamified our self-worth.

Likes. Followers. Views. Comments.

These numbers act like a scorecard for our value.

When a post performs well, we feel validated. When it doesn't, we feel invisible.

It's a digital popularity contest — one we never signed up for, but participate in anyway.

This constant measurement has led to a spike in:

- Anxiety among teens and young adults
- Declining self-esteem
- Fear of posting (aka "content paralysis")
- Obsessive checking and rechecking metrics

Even adults who think they're "too mature to care" often find themselves affected by these subtle but powerful cues.

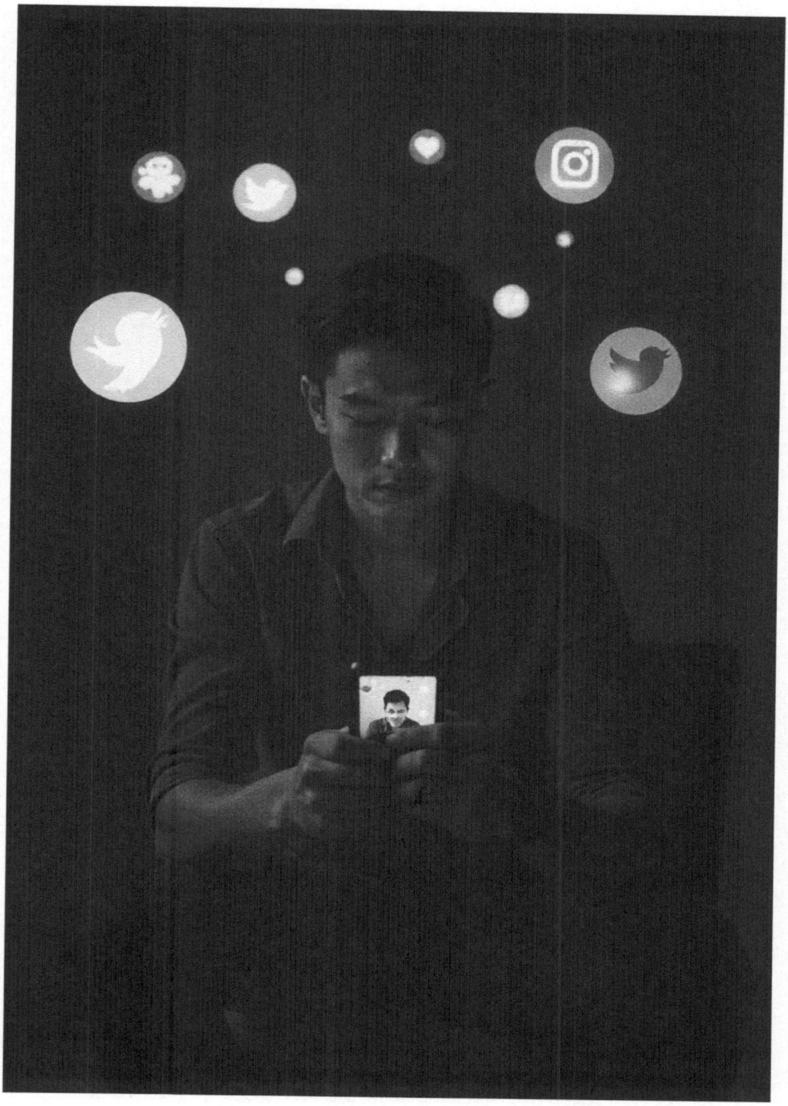

4. The Myth of Effortless Success

Social media also glamorizes something that *doesn't actually exist*: effortless success.

You'll see captions like:

- "Quit my job and made six figures in 3 months!"
- "Lost 30 pounds just by manifesting!"
- "From broke to boss babe overnight!"

But behind these stories are usually:

- Teams of marketers
- Years of failure
- Privilege, access, or inherited support
- Intense hustle that's hidden from the screen

When we buy into these myths, we feel *less than* for not achieving similar results — without knowing the real effort or circumstances behind them.

---

5. The Emotional Rollercoaster of Scrolling

Here's what a 10-minute scroll can do:

1. You see someone's wedding video → You feel lonely.
2. A friend got a promotion → You feel behind.
3. A fitness influencer shares their abs → You feel ashamed.
4. A luxury travel blogger posts a yacht video → You feel poor.

All of this — from your couch, in pajamas, after a long day of work.

You're exhausted, but now your nervous system is flooded with emotions. And the saddest part? *None of those moments had anything to do with your life.*

---

6. Real Life Is Not a Feed

Here's a grounding truth: Life isn't always pretty. It's not all aesthetic meals, dreamy vacations, and motivational quotes.

Life is:

- Missteps
- Messy rooms
- Canceled plans
- Late-night doubts
- Slow progress

And that's okay. That's what *real life* looks like.

The people who truly love you don't care about how your life *looks.* They care about how your life *feels.*

So if you're constantly chasing aesthetic perfection or online admiration, ask yourself: Is this bringing me peace — or pressure?

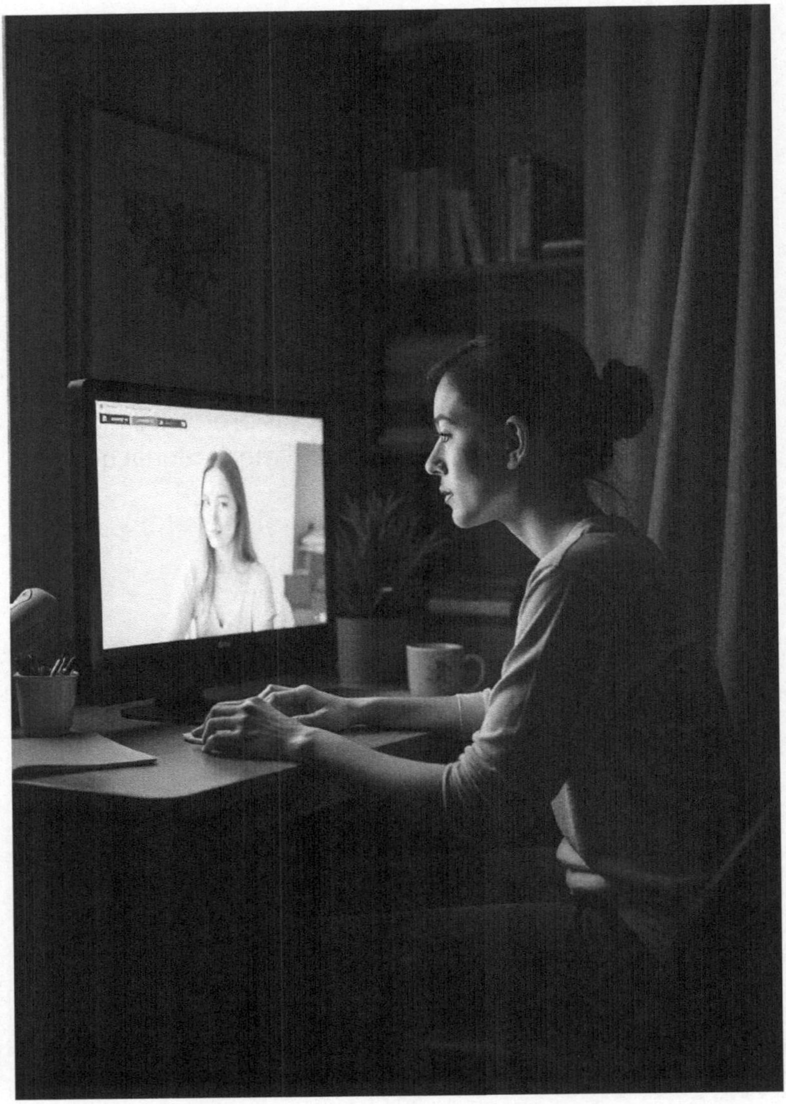

7. Breaking Free: How to Reclaim Your Joy

You don't have to quit social media — but you do need to reshape how you use it.

Here are 5 steps to help you protect your peace:

1. Curate your feed Unfollow or mute accounts that make you feel inferior, anxious, or drained. Follow people who inspire, educate, or make you laugh — without pressure.

2. Set screen-time limits Use built-in tools to limit daily usage. Less exposure = less comparison.

3. Create before you consume Start your day with something real: writing, walking, talking to a friend — *before* you open your apps.

4. Be honest online If you choose to post, let it reflect your reality. Your authenticity will encourage others to do the same.

5. Remind yourself daily:

"Their life isn't better. It's just edited."

Comparison loses its power when you reconnect with what matters to *you.*

Section 4: Creating Healthy Digital Boundaries

Let's face it — we don't live in a world without screens anymore.

From the moment we wake up to the second we shut our eyes at night, digital devices surround us. Phones, smartwatches, laptops, tablets, notifications, reminders, alerts — all vying for our attention like noisy toddlers that never nap.

And here's the thing: We're not weak for feeling overwhelmed. We're human. Our minds weren't wired to process this much stimulation 24/7. So, if we want to reclaim our calm, we don't have to quit technology — we have to build better *boundaries* with it.

That's what this section is all about.

---

1. What Are Digital Boundaries — and Why Do They Matter?

Digital boundaries are personal limits we set around our use of technology. They protect our time, focus, energy, and emotional well-being.

Think of them as fences around your mental garden.

- They keep out the digital weeds (distractions, stress, comparison).
- They help you grow what really matters (creativity, peace, presence).

Without boundaries, tech isn't just a tool — it becomes the master.

Let's shift that power back into your hands.

---

2. Start With Self-Awareness (Without Guilt)

Before setting limits, ask yourself honestly:

- When do I feel most drained after using my phone?
- What apps or platforms trigger anxiety or insecurity?
- Do I reach for my phone out of boredom, loneliness, or stress?

You're not judging yourself — you're getting to know your patterns.

Awareness isn't about blame. It's about building clarity. And clarity leads to change.

---

3. Design Your Digital Day Intentionally

Here's a fresh idea: What if your *technology* served *your life* — not the other way around?

Let's break the day into a few key zones:

Morning:

- Avoid screens for the first 30–60 minutes.
- Start with something analog: stretch, breathe, write, pray, walk.

- Give your brain space before inviting in outside noise.

Work Time:

- Use focus tools like "Do Not Disturb," Focus Mode, or website blockers.
- Batch-check emails instead of responding to each ding.
- Disable *non-essential* notifications (yes, that includes news alerts and sale offers).

Evening:

- Set a screen curfew (ideally 1 hour before sleep).
- Replace scrolling with something grounding: reading, music, journaling.
- Keep devices outside your bedroom if possible.

These aren't hard rules — they're guidelines to help you protect your mental bandwidth.

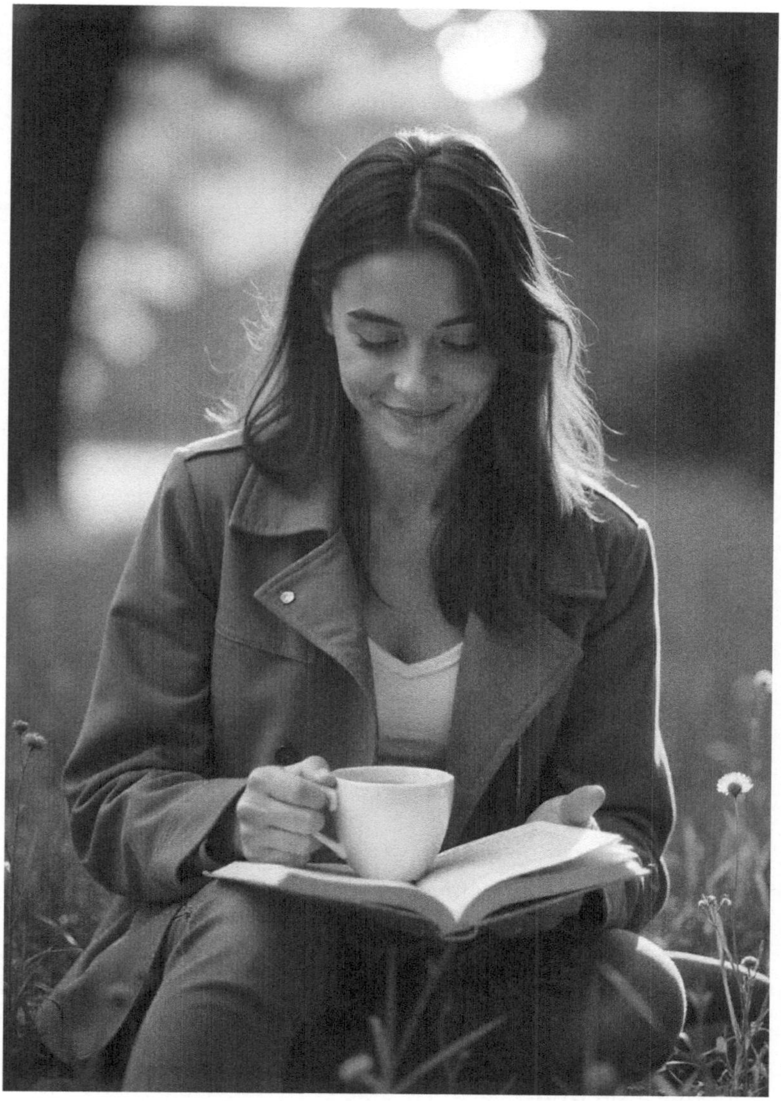

4. Use Tech to Fight Tech

Here's the ironic truth: Sometimes we need technology to help manage our relationship *with* technology.

Try these helpful apps:

- **Forest:** Stay focused by growing a virtual tree that dies if you pick up your phone.
- **Freedom or Cold Turkey:** Block distracting websites and apps.
- **Screen Time (iOS) / Digital Wellbeing (Android):** Track usage and set time limits.

You can even create automation:

- Turn Wi-Fi off at night using a smart plug.
- Schedule email checking hours.
- Set auto-replies during deep work time.

Use the tools wisely — not to punish yourself, but to protect your peace.

---

5. Redefine Urgency (Most Things Aren't)

We live in a culture of instant replies. If you don't respond to a message in five minutes, people assume something's wrong.

But here's the truth:

"Your urgency doesn't have to be my emergency."

Healthy digital boundaries include teaching others how to treat your time.

Try this:

- Set expectations with friends or coworkers: "I check my messages a few times a day."
- Use email signatures that say, "I reply within 24 hours."
- Give yourself permission to delay — and breathe.

Being always available doesn't make you more loyal, productive, or loving. It just makes you more exhausted.

Boundaries are a gift to yourself *and* others.

---

6. Create Tech-Free Zones

Some spaces deserve to be sacred.

Designate areas in your home where phones don't go:

- The dinner table → for presence and family.
- The bathroom → for hygiene and reflection.
- The bedroom → for rest and intimacy.

You'll be amazed at how powerful small pockets of disconnection can be.

Tech-free zones help retrain your brain to feel calm without constant input.

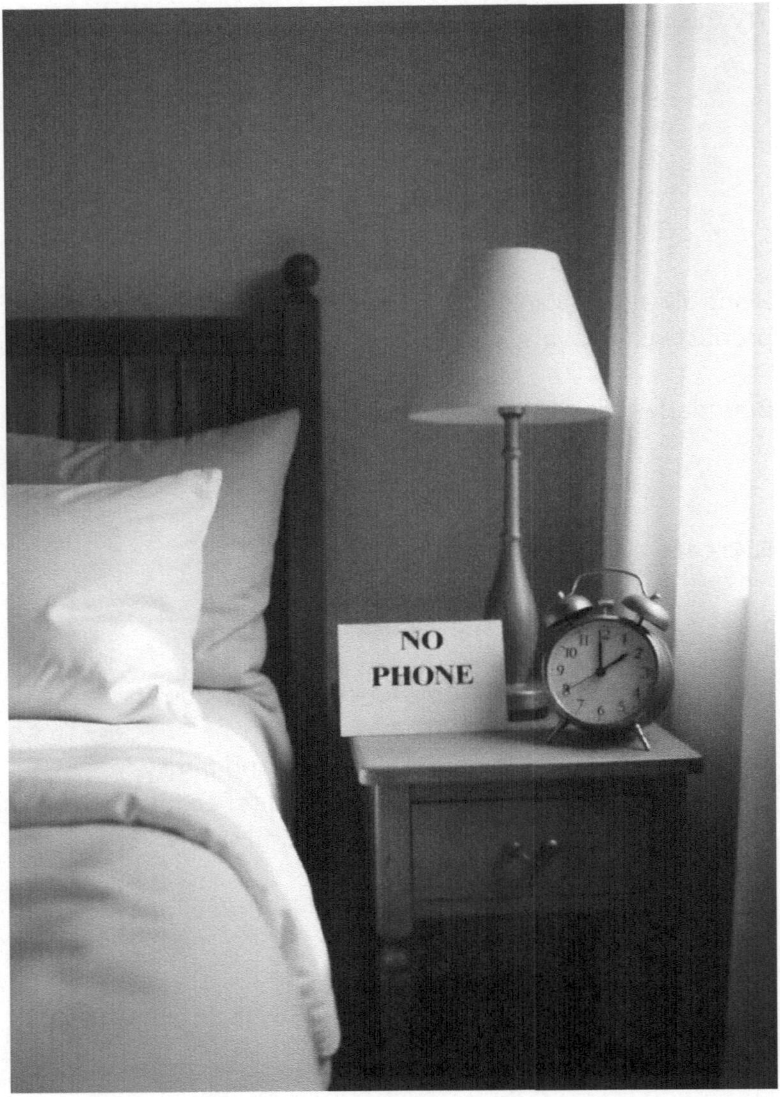
NO
PHONE

7. Practice a Digital Sabbath

Just as rest is essential for our bodies, our minds need a break from digital noise.

Try a **Digital Sabbath** once a week:

- Choose a full day or half-day to unplug.
- Let others know ahead of time.
- Plan activities that reconnect you: nature, conversation, creativity, rest.

It may feel uncomfortable at first — but you'll notice your nervous system sigh with relief.

When you step back, you regain perspective. And perspective is what anxiety steals first.

---

8. Boundaries Aren't Barriers — They're Bridges

Let's shift how we think about boundaries. They're not walls to keep people or experiences out. They're *bridges* back to our real selves.

When we set healthy limits with our devices, we:

- Show up better for our relationships.
- Reconnect with our intuition.
- Recover from overstimulation.
- Rebuild focus, peace, and presence.

Digital boundaries help us become *human again.*

They remind us that life is more than notifications, hashtags, or blue light. It's breath. It's stillness. It's connection — not through a screen, but through soul.

Section 5: Detox Without Disappearing — Small Daily Fixes

Let's be honest. When people talk about doing a "digital detox," it can sound a bit extreme.

Go offline for a week? Delete all social media? Ditch your smartphone for a flip phone? Move to the mountains with no Wi-Fi?

Sure, that works for some. But for most of us — people with jobs, responsibilities, and a genuine desire to stay connected — that's just not realistic.

Here's the good news: You don't have to disappear to reclaim your calm. You just need small, intentional daily fixes — manageable shifts that help you detox your digital habits *without* quitting modern life.

This section is about practical balance. Not tech shame. Not radical disconnection. Just gentle resets that make room for peace.

Let's dig in.

---

1. The "Mini Detox" Mindset

A detox doesn't have to mean a total shutdown.

Instead, think of it like brushing your teeth. You do it daily, not just when things get really bad.

Same with digital hygiene. Each day is a chance to:

- Clear mental clutter.
- Reconnect with what matters.
- Reduce overstimulation.
- Feel like *you* again.

Small steps can lead to major changes — without overwhelming your schedule.

---

2. The 3-Minute Reset

Start with a single moment of quiet disconnection.

Try this simple practice:

1. Put your phone in another room.
2. Sit, stand, or lie down comfortably.
3. Close your eyes and take a few slow breaths.
4. Notice what's around you: sounds, smells, sensations.
5. Stay here for three minutes.

That's it.

No apps. No scrolling. No performance.

Just you and stillness.

These short breaks teach your nervous system: "It's okay to be off. I'm still safe."

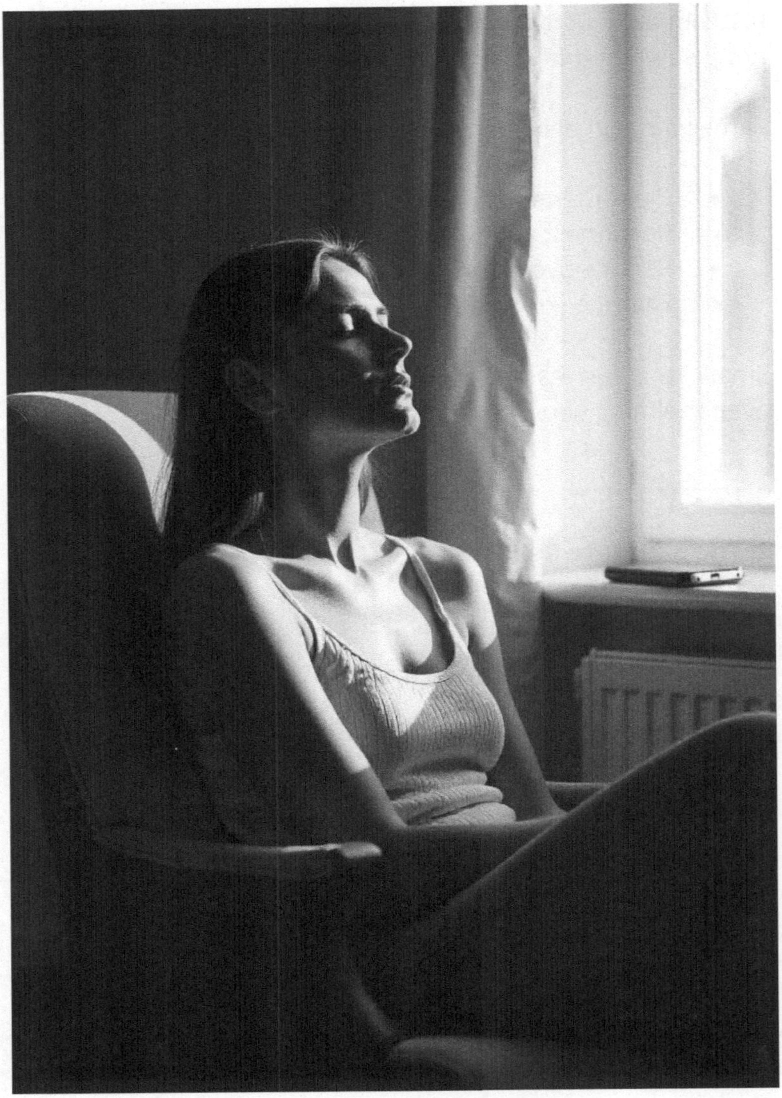

3. The One-App Rule

Try limiting yourself to using just *one social app per day* — or even one session per app.

Let's say you choose Instagram:

- Set a 10-minute timer.
- Scroll intentionally.
- Log off once the timer buzzes.

This creates a clear start and stop — and reminds your brain that social media is a tool, not a lifestyle.

You can even rotate apps. Monday: Facebook. Tuesday: Twitter. Wednesday: Pinterest.

Curate your consumption the way you'd plan a healthy meal — with awareness, not autopilot.

---

4. Build Tech-Free Anchors Into Your Day

Tech boundaries are more sustainable when they're tied to *real-life anchors*.

Some ideas:

- **Morning:** No screens until after you brush your teeth or eat breakfast.
- **Mealtimes:** Phones stay on silent and out of sight.
- **Evening:** Start a wind-down ritual: book + tea > Netflix + phone.

These moments become digital "rest stops" — giving your brain time to reset between notifications.

Bonus: You'll enjoy food, conversation, and sleep way more.

---

5. Practice the 20/20/20 Rule

This one's simple and powerful:

Every 20 minutes, look away from your screen for 20 seconds, and focus on something 20 feet away.

This not only reduces eye strain — it breaks the hyper-focus loop that leads to digital fatigue.

Set a subtle timer or sticky note as a reminder. Or use breaks to:

- Stand and stretch.
- Grab water.
- Say hello to a real human.

It's a micro-reset that builds real resilience.

---

6. Create a "Digital Landing Spot"

Designate a specific space where your devices live when they're not in use.

Maybe it's:

- A pretty tray in the entryway.
- A drawer in the kitchen.
- A charging station in the living room.

By giving your phone a home, you teach your mind: "I don't *have* to carry this with me all the time."

Out of hand = out of habit.

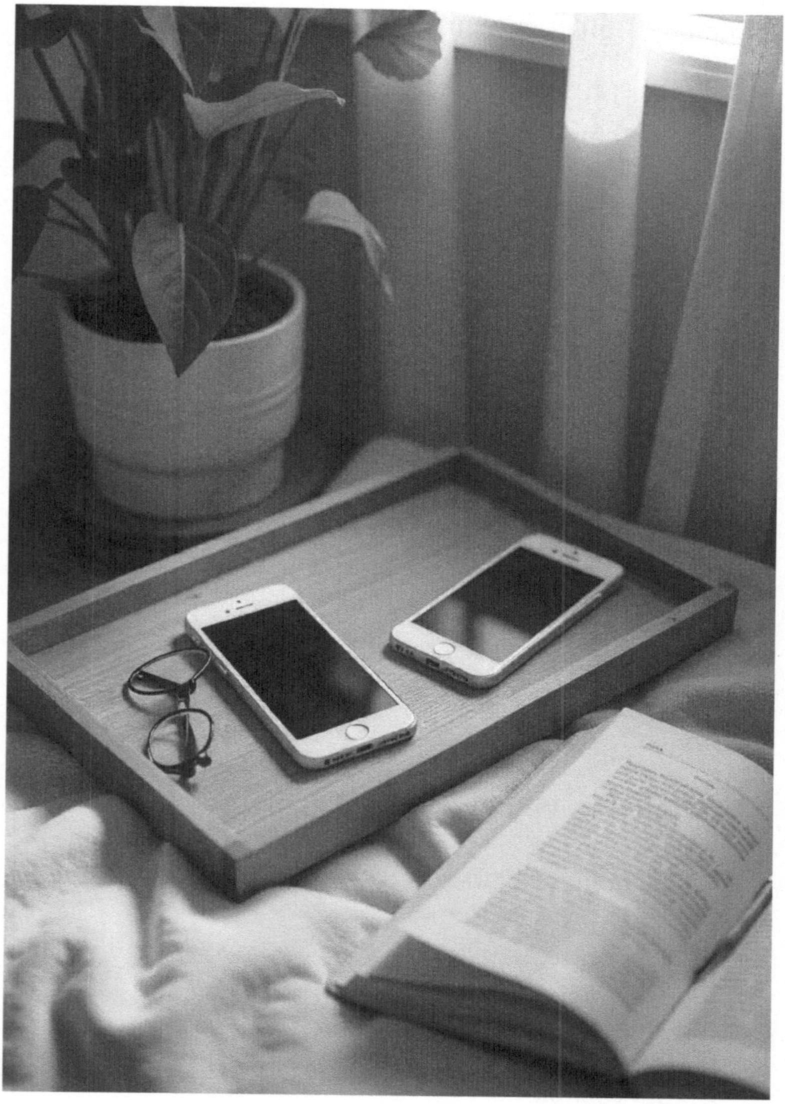

7. Replace, Don't Just Remove

Cutting down on screen time works better when you replace it with something nourishing.

Instead of just *trying not* to scroll, ask:

"What's something offline I actually enjoy?"

Ideas:

- Journaling
- Painting
- Gardening
- Playing music
- Walking
- Calling a friend (voice only!)

You're not quitting pleasure — you're rediscovering it.

---

8. End Your Day With Intention, Not Input

The last 30 minutes before sleep matter. They set the tone for your rest and the next morning.

Try:

- Reading something soothing (fiction, poetry, devotional).
- Practicing gentle breathing or prayer.
- Reflecting on 3 things you're grateful for.

Avoid:

- Breaking news
- Online debates
- Endless reels or short videos

The world can wait. Your nervous system needs the pause.

Your dreams are built on how you rest.

---

9. Digital Detox ≠ Isolation

Let's be clear — healthy tech habits don't mean ghosting your friends.

Stay connected through:

- Phone calls
- Walks together
- Voice notes instead of endless typing
- Shared hobbies

You can detox *with* your people. Invite them into the challenge. Celebrate each small shift together.

It's not about becoming a digital monk. It's about becoming a more present, peaceful version of yourself — one tap at a time.

---

10. Small Changes, Big Shifts

You don't need a big declaration to begin. You just need:

- One more mindful moment today.
- One less mindless scroll.
- One act of intentional disconnection.

These small tweaks accumulate into a life that feels lighter, calmer, more connected.

You don't need to disappear. You just need space to *reappear* — in your own life.

Let that be enough for now.

Section 6: Reclaiming Real Connection Over Virtual Clutter

Let's start with a moment of honesty. When was the last time you had a conversation—like a real, deep, eye-to-eye, belly-laugh or tear-jerking talk with someone? Not a comment thread, not a reaction emoji, not a double tap. A real conversation. If you're struggling to remember, you're not alone.

In a world more connected than ever before, we are, ironically, lonelier than ever before. The promise of the digital age was connection. And yet, here we are—anxious, overstimulated, and often emotionally isolated. But what if the connection we're so desperately scrolling for isn't lost? What if it's just buried under the clutter of constant notifications, endless feeds, and half-hearted group chats?

This section is about peeling back the noise and finding our way back to what truly connects us—real human connection. No filters. No blue ticks. Just us, talking, sharing, being present.

When Connection Becomes Consumption

Social media and digital platforms were originally meant to bring us together. And for a while, they did. We reconnected with old friends, stayed in touch with distant relatives, and found like-minded communities across the globe. But somewhere along the way, something shifted.

Now, instead of connecting, we consume. We scroll through others' lives, compare, judge, and post in the hopes of getting likes—little digital affirmations that someone, somewhere, sees us. We replace heart-to-heart talks with heart emojis. And slowly, subtly, we become more *visible* but less *known*.

Let's be clear—digital connection isn't inherently bad. In fact, it can be beautiful and life-changing when used with intention. But when it replaces real relationships rather than enhancing them, we begin to feel the ache of isolation, even in the middle of a digital crowd.

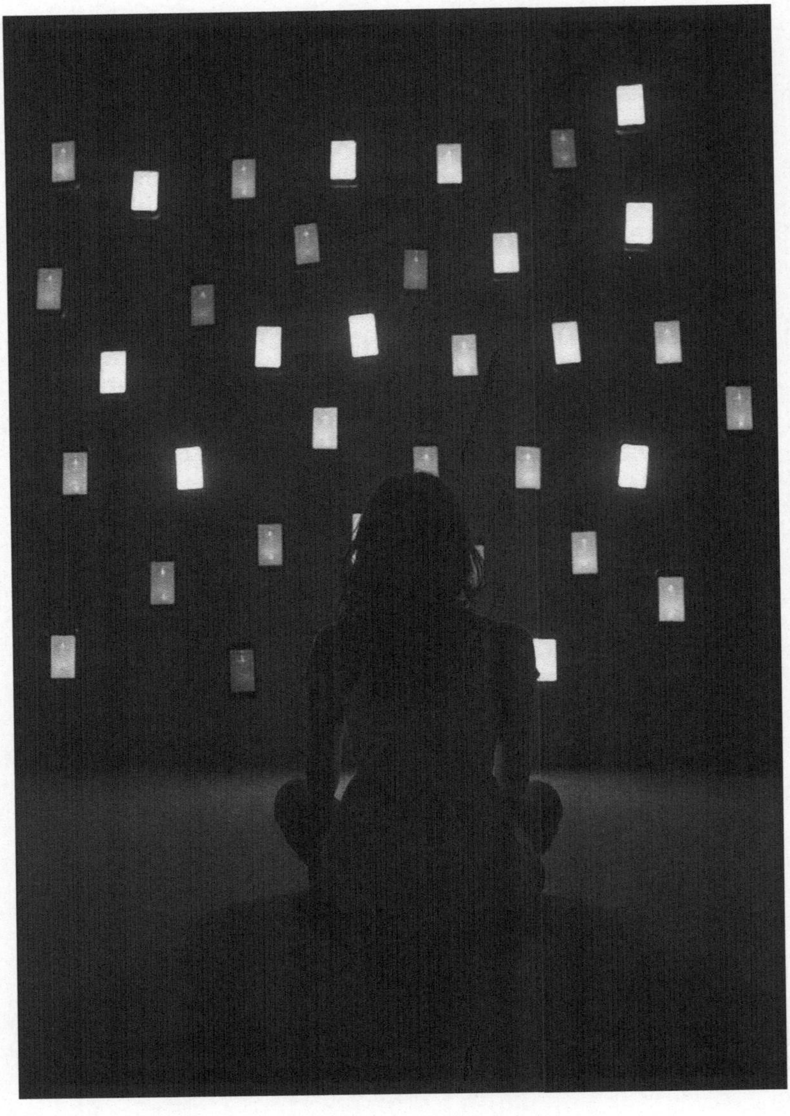

Recognizing the Real vs. the Virtual

It's important to pause and ask: *What does real connection feel like?* Chances are, it involves presence. It's unhurried. It has depth. It feels safe. And crucially, it's mutual.

Real connection happens when we:

- Listen without checking our phone
- Ask meaningful questions and wait for real answers
- Share our stories, fears, and dreams without the fear of being "unfollowed"
- Laugh until our sides hurt
- Sit in silence, and it still feels warm

On the flip side, virtual connection often becomes:

- Performance over authenticity
- Highlight reels instead of honest snapshots
- Surface-level likes over deep understanding

The difference matters. Because one nourishes your soul. The other just keeps you entertained.

Making Room for Real Moments

To reclaim real connection, we don't need to become hermits. We don't need to delete every app or disappear from the digital world. We just need to make intentional space for real-life interaction. Here's how:

1. Create "No-Phone Zones"

Designate specific times or places in your home or schedule that are tech-free. The dinner table. The first 30 minutes after you wake up. A weekly coffee with a friend. Treat these moments as sacred.

2. Practice Eye Contact

It sounds silly, but think about it: when was the last time you held eye contact during a conversation for more than five seconds without glancing at a screen? Try it. It's powerful.

3. Initiate Old-School Communication

Pick up the phone. Send a voice note. Write a letter. Organize a meet-up. Reach out just because you care—not because it's their birthday and Facebook reminded you.

4. Replace Scrolling with Sharing

Instead of doomscrolling during downtime, use that time to send a message of appreciation, encouragement, or curiosity to someone you care about. It changes everything.

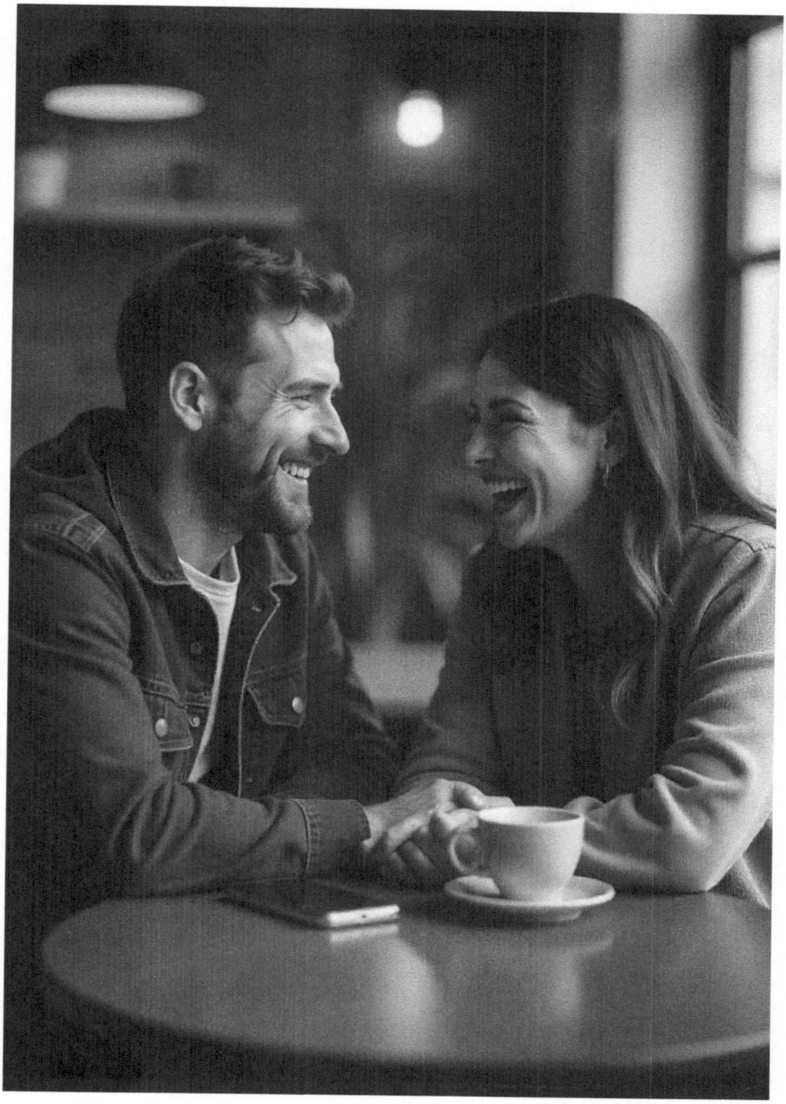

Let's Talk About Loneliness

Here's the truth that nobody wants to say out loud: loneliness isn't just an old person's problem. It's not about being physically alone. You can be in a bustling city, surrounded by hundreds of "friends" online, and still feel painfully disconnected.

Reclaiming real connection starts with acknowledging that need. It's human. It's okay. In fact, it's beautiful.

What helps?

- Vulnerability: Say "I miss you." Say "I need support."
- Being first: Don't wait for others to reach out. You take the step.
- Creating shared rituals: Weekly walks. Monthly dinners. Daily check-ins. Build rhythms that create emotional safety.

Loneliness thrives in silence. Connection thrives in shared moments—big and small.

Digital Tools Can Still Support Real Connection

This chapter isn't about demonizing technology. It's about repurposing it. We can use digital tools in ways that foster, not fracture, our relationships.

Try this:

- Create a small "inner circle" group chat for real talk
- Use calendar apps to set aside time for in-person meetings

- Curate your feed with accounts that uplift and inspire, not provoke and compare
- Use video calls to bridge long-distance relationships—but treat them like real dates. Dress up. Sit down. Be fully present.

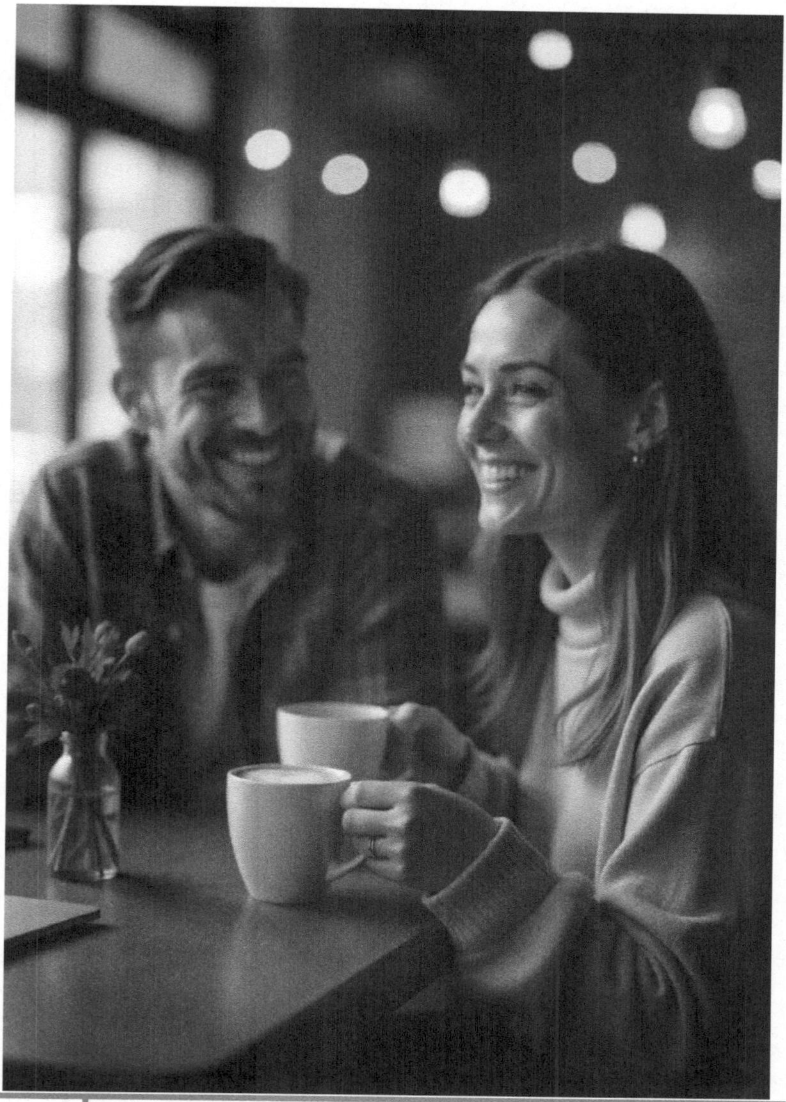

The Courage to Disconnect So You Can Reconnect

Reclaiming connection means we have to get brave. Brave enough to:

- Log off even when the conversation is "hot" online
- Say no to endless notifications
- Miss out on digital noise so we don't miss out on real presence

Because peace isn't found in the scroll. It's found in being seen, heard, and known—without the pressure to perform.

Let's not just *exist* online. Let's live, here, now, together.

Chapter 2 Summary: The Digital Drain

In this chapter, we've peeled back the shiny, seductive surface of digital life to reveal the stress, overstimulation, and isolation beneath. We explored how constant scrolling affects our nervous systems, how doomscrolling creates a fog of anxiety (aka "Techxiety"), and how comparison culture erodes our self-worth.

But we didn't stop there. We also uncovered hope:

- We can set healthy boundaries
- We can make small daily fixes without abandoning our online lives
- And most importantly, we can reconnect with what truly matters—real, human connection

The digital world is powerful—but we're more powerful when we live with intention.

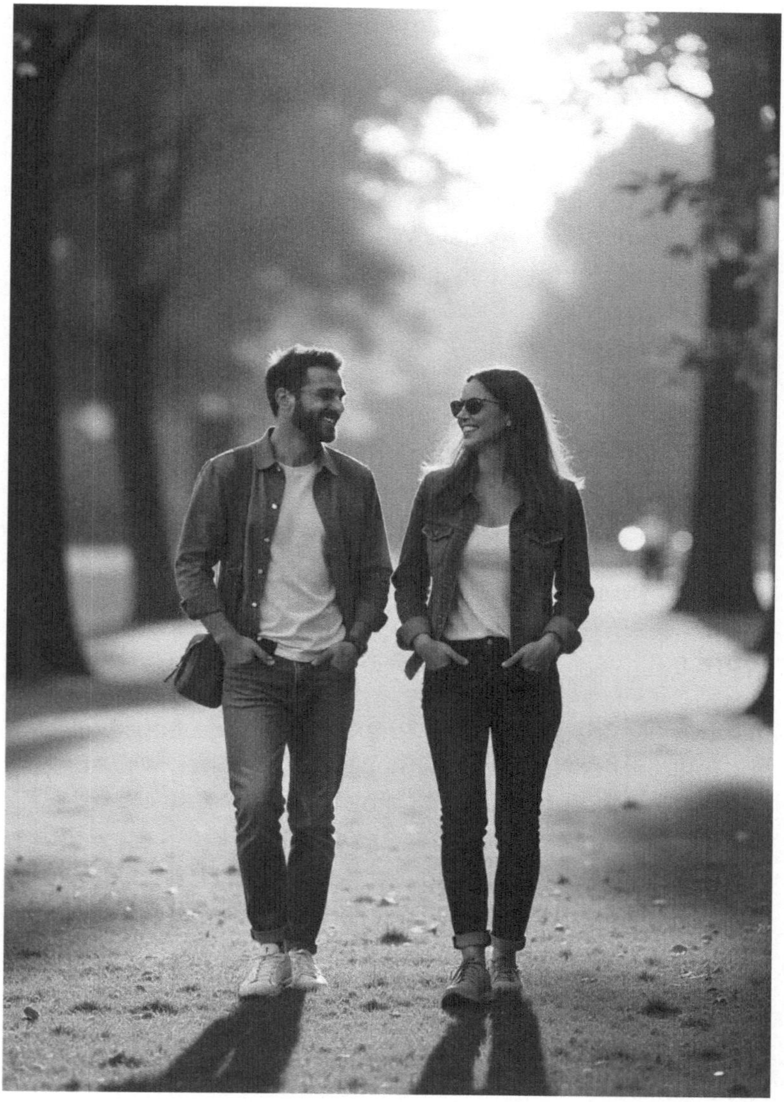

Chapter 3: Redefining Success and Slowing Down

Section 1: The Lie of Constant Productivity

Let's take a moment to be honest with ourselves. How many times have you felt like your worth is directly tied to how much you get done in a day? Whether it's checking off items on a to-do list, hitting daily fitness goals, answering every email, or "making the most" of your weekend, there's this constant pressure — unspoken but deafening — to be productive.

You wake up with your brain already racing. Your phone buzzes. There's a meeting to prep for. A project due. A social obligation looming. And somehow, through all of this, you're supposed to also meditate, eat clean, exercise, read, network, and grow your side hustle. Sound familiar?

You're not imagining it. Our world, especially in the digital age, glorifies constant productivity. From hustle culture mantras like "rise and grind" to the idolization of busy CEOs and influencers who seem to have it all together, we're surrounded by the idea that doing more is the key to being more. But let's pause for a moment: what if that's not true?

Productivity Isn't the Enemy — Perfectionism Is

There's nothing wrong with wanting to accomplish things. Being productive can feel good, fulfilling even. But when productivity becomes a measure of your identity, it quickly turns toxic.

The danger lies in the **expectation of endless output**. When rest feels like laziness, and every moment of stillness feels like time wasted, we've been sold a lie. The lie that your value as a human is tied to your ability to perform.

Perfectionism loves to disguise itself in productivity. It whispers, "If you do more, you'll finally be enough." But enough for what? For whom? And at what cost?

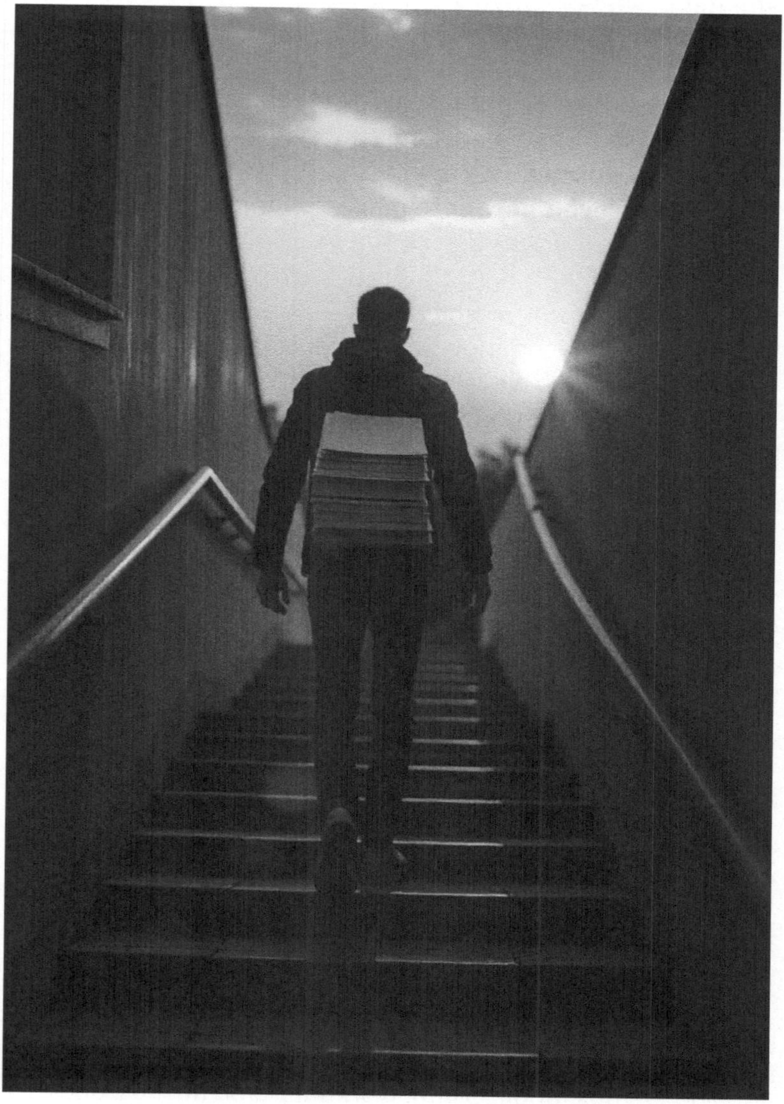

The Burnout Loop

Let's talk about burnout. It's not just exhaustion. It's deeper — emotional depletion, cynicism, and a sense of hopelessness. And yet, many of us are stuck in this loop:

1. **Push harder** because we feel behind.
2. **Crash** from exhaustion.
3. **Feel guilty** about the crash.
4. **Push even harder** to make up for lost time.

Rinse. Repeat.

This pattern is so common, we almost treat it as normal. But it's not. It's not how we're meant to live. Your body wasn't designed to sprint through life without pause.

When we don't allow ourselves moments of rest, creativity dries up, patience thins, and joy fades. Life becomes something we manage, not something we savor.

Where Did This Lie Come From?

Much of this obsession with productivity stems from cultural and economic systems that value output over wellbeing. Think about the Industrial Revolution, when labor and efficiency became the gold standard. Fast-forward to today, and we've digitized that obsession.

We wear busyness like a badge of honor. How many times have you heard (or said), "I've been so busy!" as if it's a marker of success?

Social media amplifies this by showcasing highlight reels. Influencers post about 5 a.m. workouts, side hustles, and impeccable home lives. But what's often missing is the real cost: mental health, quality relationships, and genuine rest.

Stillness Feels Unfamiliar

Here's a truth that might surprise you: *many of us are uncomfortable with stillness*. Not because it's bad, but because we're not used to it. Stillness can feel like emptiness — like we're missing out, or falling behind.

But stillness is where we reconnect with ourselves. It's in the pause that we breathe, reflect, and truly feel alive. Slowing down isn't a failure. It's a radical act of self-respect.

The Myth of Time Management

Time management gurus will tell you to wake up earlier, plan better, multitask more efficiently. And while these strategies can be helpful, they miss the deeper truth:

You don't need to manage your time better. You need to stop believing your time has to be filled to be valuable.

What if the answer isn't doing more with your time, but doing **less with more intention**?

Imagine how life might look if you:

- Prioritized deep work over busy work
- Said no to things that don't align with your values
- Allowed yourself moments of genuine rest, free from guilt
- Measured success by how you feel, not by how much you achieved

These aren't luxuries. They're essential shifts.

Redefining Success on Your Terms

One of the most freeing decisions you can make is this: **define what success means to you**.

Success doesn't have to mean climbing a corporate ladder, going viral, or hustling 24/7. Maybe success for you looks like:

- Being present with your family
- Having time to pursue hobbies that light you up
- Feeling rested when you wake up
- Cultivating peace in your heart

When you let go of the version of success someone else handed you, you start to create space for a life that actually fits *you*.

Real Talk: Slowing Down Is Scary — But Worth It

You might worry that if you slow down, you'll fall behind. That people will think you're lazy or that you won't achieve your dreams. But here's the secret: slowing down doesn't mean giving up.

It means stepping out of the hamster wheel so you can finally *run your own race*.

Your dreams still matter. But chasing them from a place of calm and clarity is much more sustainable than chasing them from burnout.

Practical Pause Practices

Let's end with a few simple ways to invite stillness into your life:

- **Tech-free mornings:** Give yourself 30 minutes after waking before checking your phone.
- **Mindful meals:** Eat without multitasking. No screens, no rush.
- **Micro-breaks:** Take 5-minute pauses between tasks to breathe, stretch, or simply sit.
- **Joy breaks:** Do something unproductive that brings you joy — doodle, dance, daydream.

These small shifts rewire your nervous system to trust that rest is not dangerous. It's nourishing.

Section 2: From Burnout to Balance: A Shift in Mindset

Let's start with something honest and possibly uncomfortable: burnout is not a badge of honor. It's not a sign that you're working hard or chasing your dreams. It's a warning light — a siren call from your body and mind that something has gone terribly off course.

Yet, so many of us wear burnout like a medal. We talk about our exhaustion with pride. We tell people how late we stayed up finishing that report or how we haven't taken a vacation in years. We believe if we're not busy — painfully busy — we must be doing something wrong. But what if the real mistake is thinking burnout is normal at all?

In this section, we're going to challenge that mindset. We're going to flip the script on what balance means, how to achieve it, and most importantly, how to give yourself permission to choose it.

The Burnout Trap

Burnout isn't just about being tired. It's chronic emotional, mental, and often physical exhaustion caused by prolonged and excessive stress. It creeps in slowly, disguising itself as ambition and responsibility. It tells you, "Just a little more," and before you know it, you're constantly running on empty.

It's not limited to career-driven professionals either. Stay-at-home parents, students, caretakers — anyone can burn out. In fact, the more you care, the more likely you are to push past your limits.

The problem? Burnout changes you. It erodes your joy, your motivation, your relationships. It makes you forget what it feels like to be well — truly, calmly, well.

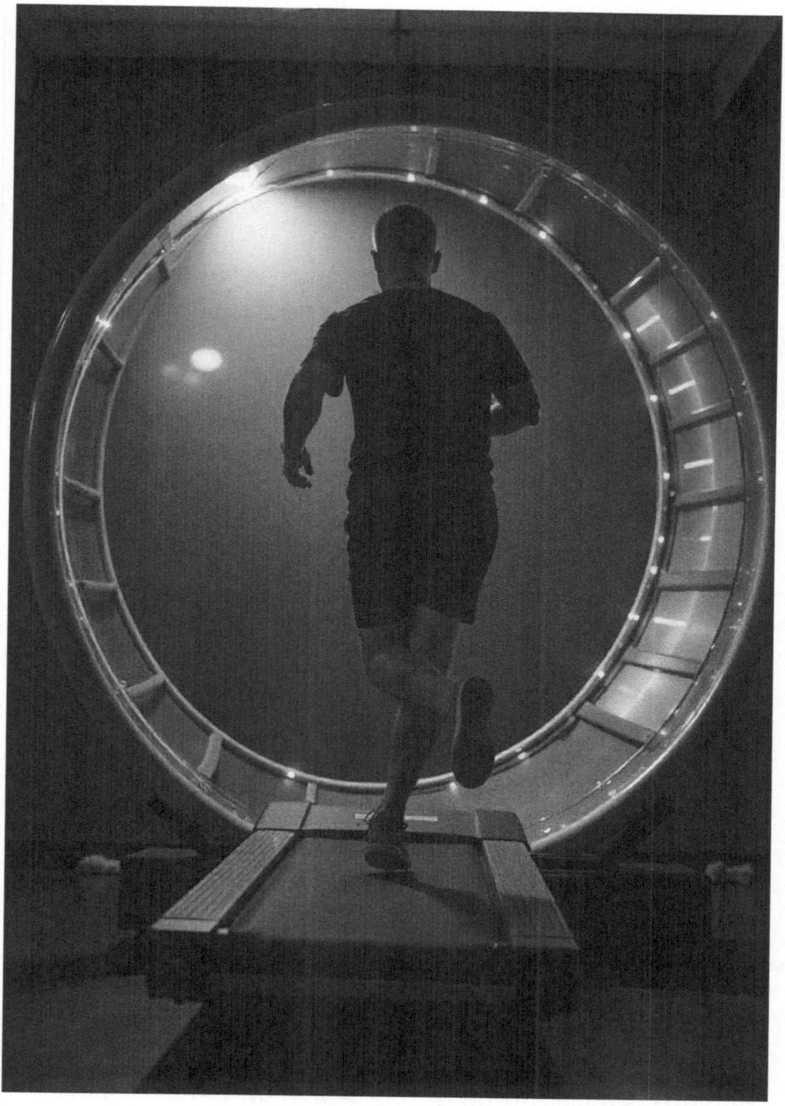

The Cost of Chronic Hustle

We've glamorized "the hustle". Entire cultures have been built on the myth that if you're not constantly producing, you're wasting time. But this ideology isn't sustainable — not for our bodies, not for our minds, and definitely not for our society.

The cost? Mental health issues. Anxiety. Depression. Lost relationships. Missed milestones. Physical illness. And ironically, decreased productivity.

Think about it. When you're overworked and burned out, are you actually doing your best work? Or are you just surviving?

When we slow down, we allow creativity, clarity, and joy to return. But the transition from hustle to harmony doesn't happen without intention.

The Balance Myth: It's Not 50/50

One common misconception about balance is that it means splitting your time and energy equally across all areas of life — work, family, self-care, social life, etc.

That's not realistic.

Real balance is fluid. It's about paying attention to what needs you most at any given moment without guilt or overcorrection. Some days, your work may demand more attention. Other days, your mental health may take priority. And sometimes, you need to drop everything and rest.

Balance is listening to your life.

How to Begin the Shift

Making the move from burnout to balance doesn't require a complete life overhaul overnight. It starts with small, powerful shifts in mindset:

1. **Stop romanticizing exhaustion.** Busy is not a personality trait. Your worth is not tied to your schedule.
2. **Redefine productivity.** What if being productive meant restoring your energy, nurturing relationships, and pursuing joy?
3. **Say no to things that drain you.** Even if you used to love them. Even if someone else expects you to do them. You can't pour from an empty cup.
4. **Celebrate rest.** Sleep, silence, solitude — these are not luxuries. They are foundational.
5. **Practice 'one thing' thinking.** Instead of doing five things halfway, do one thing well. Then move on to the next.

These shifts are not selfish. They're survival. They're the soil in which a healthy, calm, and meaningful life can grow.

Real Life: Meet Olivia

Olivia was a marketing executive in New York. Her days were a blur of meetings, metrics, and managing a team. She loved her job — or thought she did. Slowly, she stopped sleeping well, felt emotionally numb, and dreaded Monday mornings more than ever.

It wasn't until Olivia fainted at work and was rushed to the ER that she realized something had to change.

What saved her wasn't quitting her job (she didn't). It was redefining how she approached her life.

She scheduled breaks. She protected her evenings. She stopped checking email after 7 p.m. She picked up painting — just for fun, no pressure. Six months later, her health improved, her team noticed her renewed energy, and for the first time in years, she felt in control.

The takeaway? You don't have to abandon your life to escape burnout. You just need to take the wheel again.

Practices for Balance

Here are a few grounded, practical things you can try today:

- **The 3-2-1 Rule Before Bed:** 3 hours before bed, no food. 2 hours before bed, no work. 1 hour before bed, no screens.
- **The 5-Minute Reset:** Set a timer. Close your eyes. Breathe deeply. Just five minutes — no scrolling, no planning, no pressure.
- **Schedule white space.** Literally add "Do Nothing" to your calendar once a week.
- **Journal your energy.** Track what activities drain you and what fills you. Make changes accordingly.

These aren't magic bullets. But over time, they nudge your brain out of survival mode and into something much more sustainable.

Mindset Mantras to Hold On To

Write these down. Post them on your mirror. Speak them when you forget:

- "I am allowed to rest."
- "My worth is not measured by my output."
- "Balance is not a luxury; it's a necessity."
- "Slow is not lazy. Slow is wise."

Burnout is loud, but balance is powerful. It speaks softly at first — in moments of peace, in clarity of thought, in better sleep and stronger relationships. If you listen, it grows louder. And one day, you wake up and realize you're living a life that feels like your own.

So here's your challenge: Don't wait for a breakdown to pursue balance. Let this be your turning point — from burnout to something better.

Let's keep walking this journey together.

Section 3: Why "Rest" Isn't Laziness

We live in a world that glorifies hustle. There's a popular saying, "You can sleep when you're dead." People wear their exhaustion like a badge of honor, as if being burned out proves they're committed, strong, and successful. But let's pause here. What if everything we've been taught about rest is wrong? What if rest isn't the opposite of ambition but the very fuel for it?

The Cultural Narrative: Rest Equals Weakness

From a young age, many of us internalize the idea that rest is something you earn after proving yourself. We see the stories of entrepreneurs pulling all-nighters, students drinking cup after cup of coffee just to keep going, and parents juggling five things at once with no break in sight. The common theme? If you stop, you're falling behind. If you rest, you must not be trying hard enough.

This belief system is deeply rooted in both Western and Eastern cultures in different ways. In the West, productivity is often tied to personal value. In the East, the sacrifice of self for family or duty is deeply admired. In both cases, rest becomes a luxury or even a sign of failure.

But here's the truth: **rest is not laziness**. It is a biological, emotional, and psychological necessity. And choosing to rest doesn't make you weak — it makes you wise.

The Physiology of Rest

Let's talk science for a moment. Our bodies and brains are not machines. Even machines need to be powered off or rebooted. Our nervous system, particularly the parasympathetic nervous system, activates during periods of rest. It helps our body recover, heal, digest food properly, and process emotions.

When we deny ourselves rest, we flood our systems with stress hormones like cortisol and adrenaline. Over time, this can lead to anxiety, depression, weakened immunity, heart issues, and chronic fatigue. It's not just that rest is good for you — not resting is *bad* for you.

Consider sleep, one of the purest forms of rest. Even losing just a few hours a night can impair memory, concentration, and mood. Yet sleep is often the first thing we sacrifice when life gets busy.

Redefining Productivity

Here's a radical idea: **True productivity includes rest**.

High performers in every industry — athletes, musicians, CEOs — know that rest is part of the process. It's during downtime that the brain consolidates information, finds creative solutions, and restores energy. Athletes take recovery days seriously. Musicians rest their hands and minds. So why do we think we're above that?

Imagine a world where your to-do list includes "take a nap," "go for a walk," or "unplug and read for pleasure." This isn't laziness; it's strategic living. It's choosing sustainability over short-term sprints.

Try This Exercise: Write down three activities that genuinely help you feel rested (not scrolling on your phone!). Schedule them into your calendar this week like you would a meeting or deadline. Give rest priority.

The Mental Load and Invisible Exhaustion

Especially for caregivers, parents, and those in emotionally taxing roles, the mental load can be staggering. Planning meals, remembering birthdays, managing everyone's schedules — it's a hidden burden that rarely gets acknowledged, let alone rested.

For these groups, rest isn't just a break from physical labor. It's a break from *thinking* about everything for everyone else. Mental rest might look like:

- A quiet drive alone
- Listening to music
- Sitting in silence
- Taking a bath

Let's honor those forms of rest. They may not be Instagram-worthy, but they are soul-saving.

Breaking the Guilt Cycle

Many people say, "I feel guilty when I rest." If that's you, you're not alone. The guilt comes from years of conditioning. But what if you could flip the narrative?

Instead of asking, "Do I deserve to rest?" try asking, "How much better will I be — for myself and others — when I'm rested?"

Because here's the thing: Rested people make better decisions. They're kinder, more focused, more creative. Rest isn't selfish — it's generous.

Real-Life Example: Sarah, a mother of three and full-time teacher, used to work until midnight every night grading papers. She felt like a failure if she watched TV or read a novel. But after burning out and getting sick, she began scheduling just 30 minutes of reading time for herself each night. Not only did her sleep improve, but her mood, patience, and classroom performance did too.

The Spiritual and Emotional Side of Rest

In many religious traditions, rest is sacred. In the Christian tradition, even God rested on the seventh day. In Judaism, the Sabbath is a dedicated day of rest. In Islam, moments of prayer punctuate the day, offering rhythm and reflection. In Buddhism, meditation is a practice of mindful rest.

Rest reconnects us with ourselves. It brings us back to our bodies, our breath, our values. It helps us notice what we're feeling instead of pushing it aside. Without rest, we lose the ability to hear our own inner wisdom.

Making Rest Part of Everyday Life

The good news? Rest doesn't require a vacation or a weekend away. It can be woven into the smallest parts of your day:

- Drinking your coffee without multitasking
- Taking three deep breaths between meetings
- Turning your phone off for 15 minutes
- Saying "no" when you need to

These micro-moments add up. They signal to your brain and body that you are safe, cared for, and allowed to slow down.

Final Thought: Rest Is Resistance

In a culture that says, "You are only as good as what you produce," choosing rest is a revolutionary act. It says, "I am worthy, even when I'm still." It reclaims your humanity in a system that wants you to be a machine.

You don't have to wait until you're burned out to give yourself rest. You can build it in now — not as a reward for doing everything, but as a foundation for doing anything well.

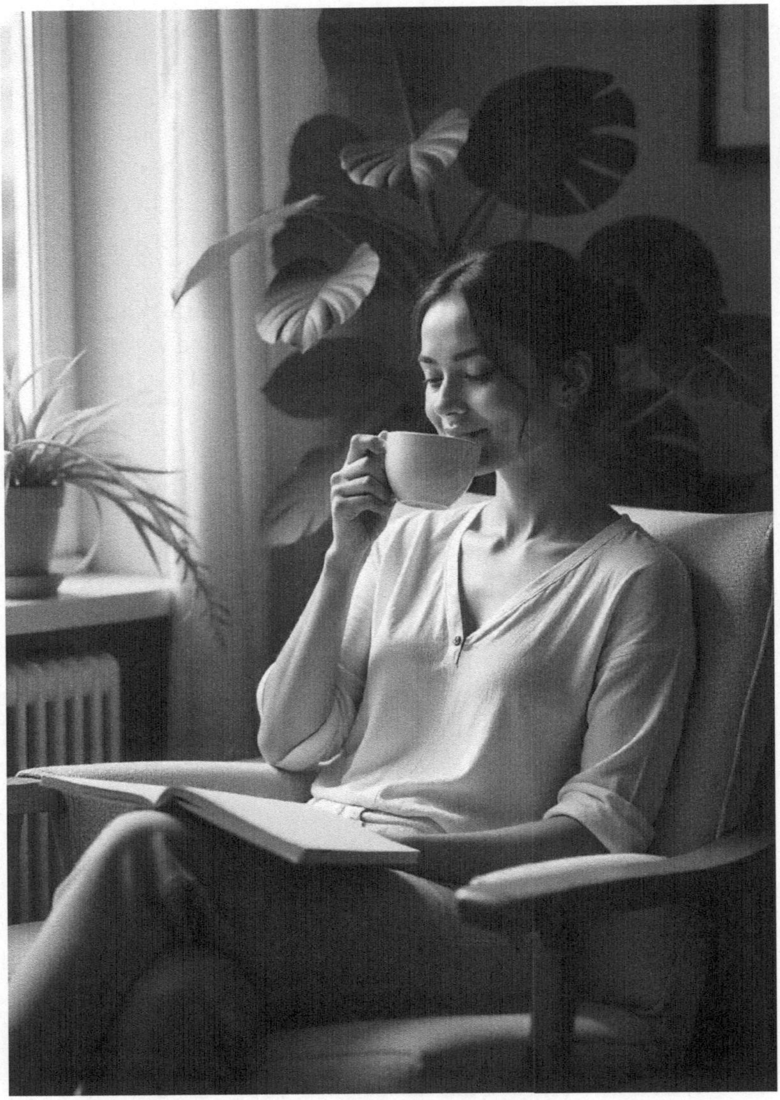

Section 4: Embracing Slow Living in a Fast World

Let's be honest: slowing down can feel almost rebellious.

In a world where busy is celebrated and burnout is worn like a badge of honor, choosing a slower pace often comes with raised eyebrows. We're so used to rushing through life — emails, errands, meetings, texts, scrolling — that doing anything slowly feels...wrong. But here's a radical truth: Slow living isn't about doing less; it's about doing what matters with more presence.

Slow living is not about laziness, denial of ambition, or isolating yourself on a farm with zero Wi-Fi (unless that's your dream). It's a conscious lifestyle that says, "I refuse to live on autopilot." It's about reclaiming moments that matter and creating a rhythm that nourishes your soul instead of draining it.

Let's explore how slow living can be a gentle rebellion that brings clarity, calm, and purpose back into your everyday life.

What Is Slow Living, Really?

Slow living is an intentional approach to life. It means making choices that prioritize quality over quantity — depth over speed. Instead of constantly reacting, it's about responding thoughtfully. You're not sprinting through the day with a to-do list clenched in your teeth — you're walking with purpose, even if the world seems to be running.

At its heart, slow living is:

- Living mindfully and with awareness

- Being present with your food, your work, your loved ones, and your own thoughts
- Choosing simplicity over noise
- Creating space in your schedule and soul

It doesn't mean you abandon modern life. It means you get to define how modern life looks for you.

The Fast Life Illusion

Why do we glorify the hustle?

Because we've been conditioned to believe that speed equals success. If you're busy, you must be important. If your calendar is full, you must be productive. If your phone is buzzing constantly, you must be needed.

But underneath that fast-paced exterior often lies:

- Anxiety
- Sleep deprivation
- Decision fatigue
- Shallow relationships
- Creative exhaustion

You don't have to be "on" 24/7 to be valuable. You don't have to constantly hustle to have worth. The fast life gives the illusion of control while often robbing us of depth and fulfillment.

How Slow Living Can Change Everything

When you begin to slow down, surprising things happen:

- **You start to notice more.** The sound of birds. The taste of fresh fruit. The warmth of sunlight.

- **You become more grounded.** Less distracted, less reactive.
- **You rediscover joy in the small.** Folding laundry while listening to music. Cooking dinner without rushing. Walking slowly and breathing deeply.
- **You reconnect with yourself.** With your values, dreams, limits, and true desires.

You may even find that productivity increases — not because you're doing more, but because you're focused, rested, and aligned.

Global Voices: How the World Is Slowing Down

Around the world, people are embracing the slow life:

- In **Sweden**, the concept of *lagom* promotes balance and moderation in everything — not too much, not too little.
- In **Italy**, the *slow food movement* was born to honor local cuisine, traditions, and the joy of cooking and eating mindfully.
- In **Japan**, *ikigai* (reason for being) emphasizes a life of meaning and alignment.
- In **India**, ancient yogic practices remind us of stillness, breath, and presence as paths to inner peace.

Slow living isn't a trend. It's a return. A return to living as humans were meant to — with connection, with rhythm, with care.

Small Ways to Start Living Slower

You don't need to quit your job, sell all your stuff, or move to a mountaintop to live more slowly. Start where you are. Choose a few gentle changes and let them ripple outward.

Here are practical ways to embrace slow living today:

- **Start your day without a screen.** Give yourself 15 minutes in the morning for silence, reflection, or stretching.
- **Savor meals.** Eat without multitasking. Notice the flavors. Chew slowly. Express gratitude.
- **Simplify your schedule.** Say no more often. Prioritize what truly matters.
- **Embrace analog moments.** Write in a journal. Read a physical book. Take a tech-free walk.
- **Add buffers between appointments.** Stop cramming your calendar.
- **Practice monotasking.** Focus on one thing at a time. Your brain will thank you.
- **Spend time in nature.** Even 10 minutes under a tree can shift your nervous system.

Slow living doesn't require perfection. It requires permission — from yourself.

The Emotional Benefits of Slowing Down

Slowing down isn't just a logistical shift. It's emotional and spiritual.

When we slow down:

- We **breathe deeper** — both literally and metaphorically.
- We **feel more grounded** — not scattered.
- We **regain control** — not by doing more, but by doing less that matters more.
- We **break free from comparison** — because we're no longer racing anyone.

Slow living becomes a kind of therapy — a healing space in your everyday life.

When Slow Feels Uncomfortable

If slowing down feels hard, that's okay. Many of us are so used to rushing that stillness feels like idleness. But stillness is where insight lives. Don't judge yourself if slowing down feels awkward at first — it's a transition.

It takes courage to shift gears in a speeding world.

Try saying:

"I'm not falling behind. I'm returning to myself."

Let that be your mantra when fear of slowing rises up.

You Deserve a Life That Feels Like Yours

At the end of the day, slow living is about alignment. It's about building a life that feels like it belongs to you — not your job, your calendar, your social media feed, or someone else's expectations.

If the life you're living feels like a blur, this is your invitation to slow down and rewrite the pace. Not because it's trendy, but because peace is your birthright.

Let the world race. You can choose stillness. You can reclaim rhythm. You can rediscover joy.

That's not just slow living — that's *real living*.

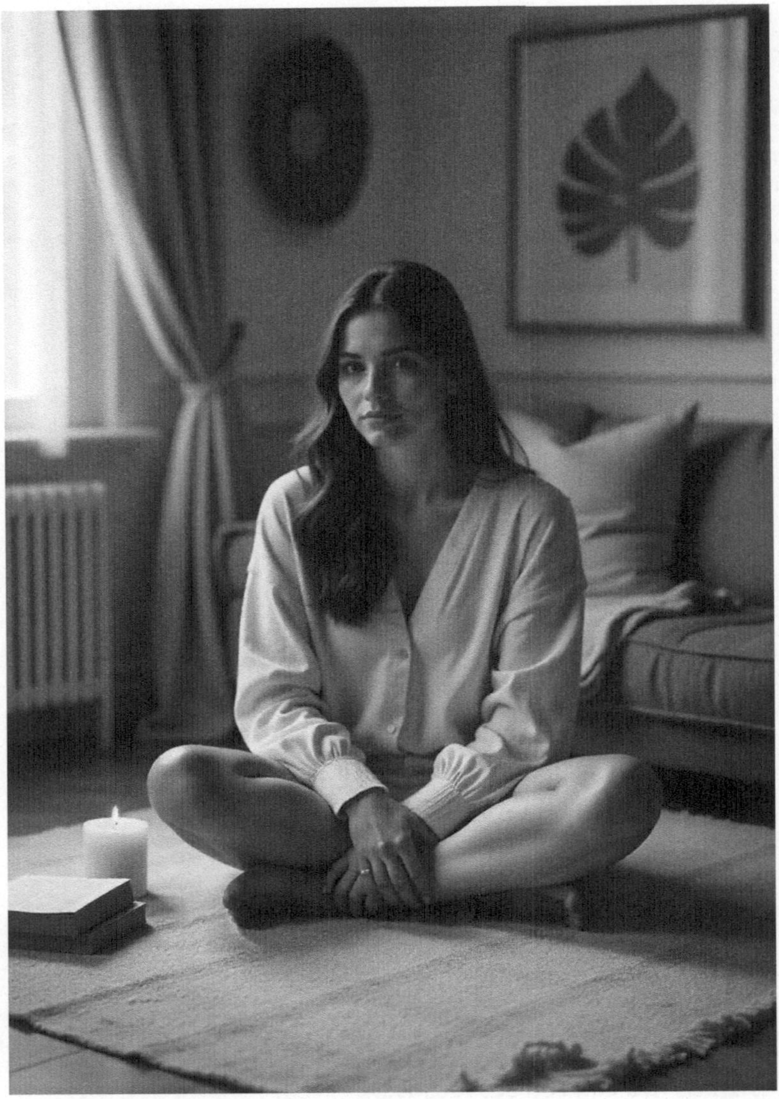

Section 5: Learning to Say "No" Without Guilt

Let's be honest: saying "no" can feel like a betrayal. We've grown up in a world that praises the yes-sayers — the people-pleasers, the go-getters, the always-available multitaskers. Somewhere along the way, we internalized the idea that our worth is tied to how much we do and how much we give to others — even if it drains us. But if we want to reclaim our calm, reset our priorities, and live authentically, we must learn the sacred power of saying "no" — without guilt.

This isn't about being selfish. It's about being sane.

The Cultural Conditioning of Saying "Yes"

From an early age, we are praised when we're helpful, agreeable, and accommodating. "Good boy." "Good girl." "Such a team player."

While these affirmations were meant to encourage kindness, they often taught us that agreeing to everything — even at the cost of our well-being — is what makes us lovable. This lesson morphs into adulthood, where we say yes to overtime we don't want, social events we dread, and favors that stretch us thin, all because we're afraid of disappointing someone or being seen as lazy, ungrateful, or uncooperative.

The truth? Every time we say yes to something that isn't aligned with our values or capacity, we are saying no to something that is. Often, that "something" is rest, peace, family time, self-respect, or space for what truly matters.

The Internal Tug-of-War: Why Saying No Feels So Hard

Saying "no" taps into emotional vulnerabilities. You might fear:

- **Rejection**: "What if they get upset or leave me out next time?"
- **Judgment**: "They'll think I'm not capable or helpful."
- **Guilt**: "I should be able to handle this. I feel bad turning them down."
- **Fear of missed opportunities**: "What if this is my only shot?"

These fears are valid. But they don't need to control your decisions. Boundaries are not walls — they are gates. They don't shut people out; they protect what's sacred within.

Reframing "No" as a Positive Act

Let's flip the narrative. Saying "no" isn't a rejection — it's a redirection.

When you say "no" to what doesn't serve you, you make space for:

- Deeper rest
- More intentional relationships
- Meaningful work
- Mental clarity
- Spiritual alignment

This kind of "no" is not reactive — it's intentional. It's a declaration that you value your time, energy, and health.

Examples of positive redirection:

- Saying no to a draining social event and instead spending the evening with your kids
- Declining a last-minute work request to honor a pre-scheduled personal retreat
- Turning down a collaboration that doesn't align with your purpose or passion

You're not rejecting people. You're honoring yourself.

Scripts for Saying "No" With Grace

Saying "no" doesn't have to be dramatic or harsh. The goal is to be clear, kind, and confident. Here are some real-life, human-style scripts you can use:

1. **Simple and direct**:
   "Thanks for thinking of me, but I can't commit to this right now."
2. **Affirming your limits**:
   "I'm already at capacity, and I wouldn't be able to give this the energy it deserves."
3. **Redirecting kindly**:
   "That's not something I can do, but I'd be happy to recommend someone else who might be a fit."
4. **Personal time matters**:
   "I've blocked that day for rest/family/personal time, and I'm keeping that commitment."

The magic happens when you practice these lines and make them your own. Your confidence will grow with every "no" you give that reflects your truth.

The Empowering Results of Healthy Boundaries

When you begin to say "no" without guilt:

- You stop overcommitting and resenting others
- You experience more peace and balance
- Your relationships become more authentic — based on truth, not performance
- You have more time for what really fuels you
- You inspire others to honor their own limits

Most importantly, you begin to trust yourself again. You no longer say yes just to avoid tension — you say yes when you mean it.

And here's a hidden bonus: when you say "no" to the wrong things, the right things begin to show up. The invitations that honor your time. The relationships that respect your energy. The opportunities that align with your purpose.

That's the deeper power of "no." It's a gateway to a more grounded, calm, and intentional life.

A Quick Boundary Checklist

Before agreeing to something, ask:

- Does this align with my priorities?
- Will I resent doing this later?
- Am I saying yes just to avoid guilt?
- What will I need to give up to say yes to this?

Let these questions be your guide. They're not about being selfish — they're about being mindful.

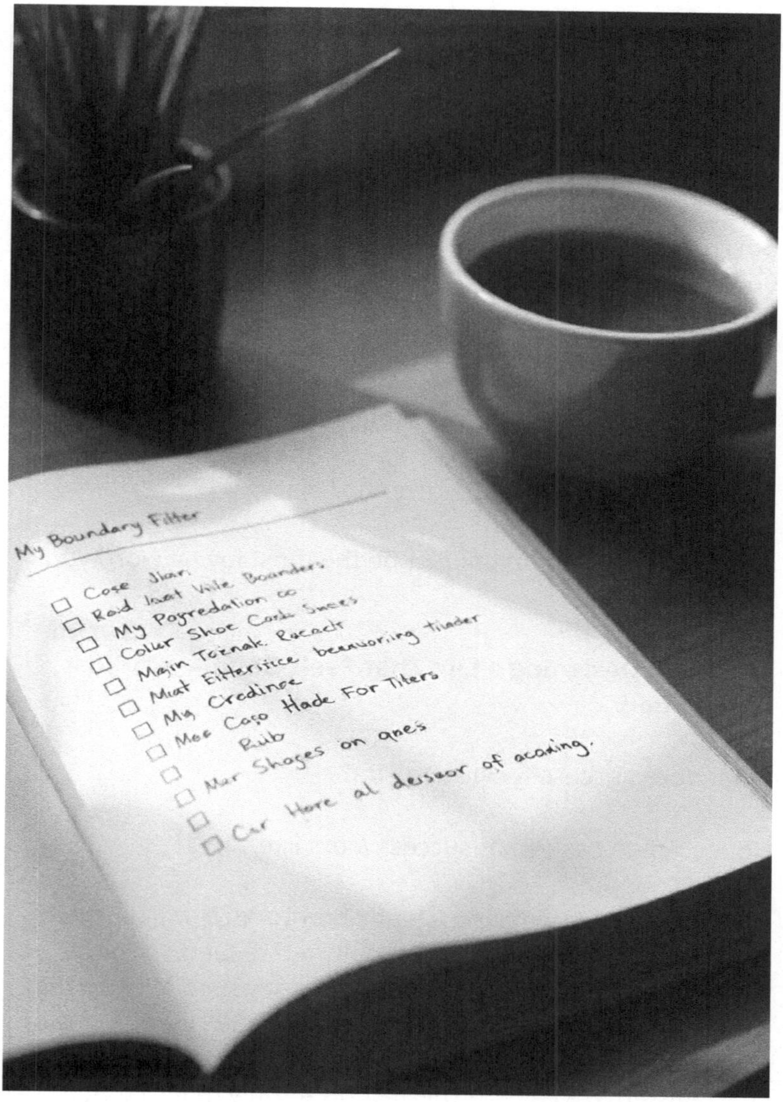
My Boundary Filter

Final Words: "No" as an Act of Self-Compassion

Learning to say "no" is like learning a new language. It's awkward at first. You might stumble. You'll over-apologize or second-guess yourself. That's okay.

But the more you speak this truth, the more fluent you become in the language of peace.

You deserve a life that doesn't drain you. One where your worth isn't measured by how much you produce or please. One where you get to be present, joyful, and whole.

It all begins with a single, brave "no."

And that "no"? That might just be the most loving word you say today.

Section 6: Designing a Life That Feels Good — Not Just Looks Good

What does success feel like to you?

Notice, I didn't ask what success *looks* like.

In a world where we're constantly bombarded with curated highlight reels on social media, polished résumés, glossy LinkedIn updates, and lifestyle vlogs, it's easy to fall into the trap of *performing* success instead of *experiencing* it. Many of us build lives based on what we think will impress others — chasing status, wealth, or perfection — only to find that it leaves us drained, discontent, and disconnected from who we truly are.

This section is your invitation to change that.

Let's talk about creating a life that's meaningful, fulfilling, and emotionally nourishing — one that feels right in your soul, not just in your Instagram feed.

The Mask of Appearances

There's a silent pressure to look like we've got it all together. Whether it's the perfect family portrait, an envy-worthy career, or a beautiful home, we often craft a persona that fits society's mold of what a successful life should look like. But what happens when that life feels like a costume we wear instead of a reflection of who we are?

The truth is, outward appearances don't always match internal realities. A person can look accomplished but feel empty. They can smile in photos and cry when they're alone. They can have every box ticked off — career, marriage, kids, house — and still wonder, *Is this it?*

We need to stop designing our lives to win applause and start designing them to feel like home.

Listening to Your Inner Compass

Designing a life that feels good starts with one essential shift: tuning into your own voice instead of everyone else's.

What lights you up? What makes you feel calm? Where do you feel most like yourself?

Many of us don't pause long enough to ask these questions, let alone answer them. We've been taught to chase dreams that weren't even ours to begin with — expectations from parents, culture, or society. But when you start asking these questions honestly, something beautiful happens. You begin to realign with your values, passions, and rhythms.

This is where peace lives — not in reaching the next milestone, but in *living* aligned with what really matters to you.

The Cost of a Shiny Life

A life built only to impress others often comes at a hidden cost:

- Chronic stress from always having to keep up appearances
- Shallow relationships based on image, not authenticity
- Fatigue from chasing goals that never feel quite satisfying
- A constant fear of being found out as someone who *doesn't* have it all together

The cost is high. The reward? Fleeting approval.

Let that sink in: We trade lasting peace for temporary praise.

And the scariest part? We can spend years — even decades — chasing something that never belonged to us. That's not failure; it's misdirection. The good news is, no matter how long you've been on the wrong road, you can turn around today.

Your New Blueprint for Living

So what does a life that *feels good* look like?

Here are a few clues:

- You wake up without dread because your days aren't packed with obligations you secretly hate.
- Your relationships are honest, raw, and real — not just performative.
- You create space for rest, reflection, and things that restore your energy.
- You define success by how you *feel*, not just how much you've achieved.
- You value slow moments and meaningful conversations over constant hustle.

This doesn't mean life will be perfect. But it will be *yours*. And that makes all the difference.

Exercise: Take a piece of paper and draw two columns. Label one: "Things that impress others." Label the other: "Things that bring me joy."

Now fill in both lists.

You may be surprised at how different they look.

Real Stories, Real Shifts

Let's look at two short global stories:

1. Lara, Sweden – From Burnout to Beekeeping
Lara worked as a high-level executive for over 12 years. Her lifestyle was glamorous but exhausting. After a health scare, she quit her job and started a small beekeeping business in the countryside. Today, she earns less — but sleeps better, smiles more, and finally feels connected to life.

2. Arjun, India – Redefining Family Priorities
Arjun was a tech consultant in Bangalore. He found himself constantly traveling, working weekends, and missing precious moments with his young daughter. He took a less demanding remote role, moved closer to extended family, and started coaching cricket on weekends. His life is simpler — but fuller.

These aren't just inspiring anecdotes. They're reminders that fulfillment isn't found in *more* — it's found in *meaning*.

Designing YOUR Version of Enough

Here's a radical thought: What if your life didn't need to be impressive to anyone else but you?

You don't have to be a minimalist or quit your job to make meaningful change. Maybe it's about:

- Setting clear work-life boundaries
- Choosing presence over perfection
- Cutting out commitments that drain you
- Letting go of goals that no longer serve you

Designing a life that feels good is about choosing what to carry — and what to release. It's not about abandoning ambition, but about grounding it in peace and authenticity.

You get to define what "enough" looks like. Not your neighbor. Not social media. Not your old self from five years ago.

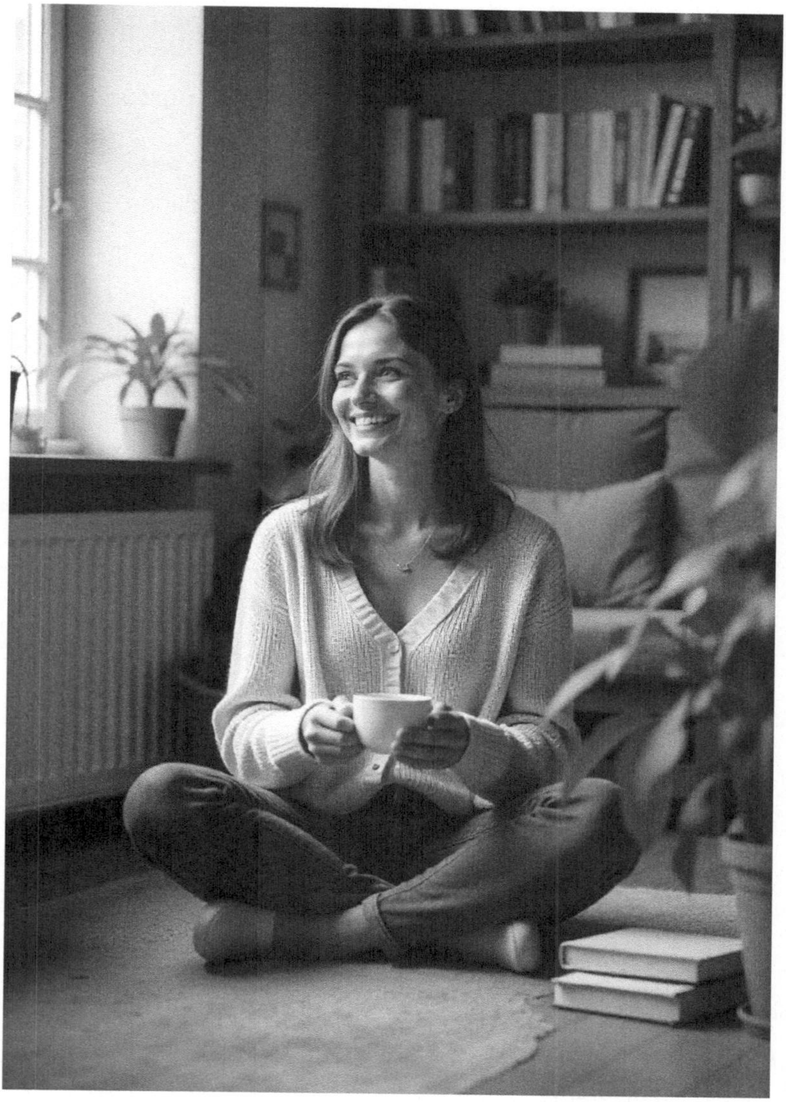

Let Peace Be the Measure

Here's your permission slip: You are allowed to pursue a life that brings peace to your mind and heart.

It might not win awards. It might not make headlines. But it will let you exhale.

When you strip away the noise and distractions, what remains? If it feels grounded, authentic, and good to your soul — that's your path.

The outer world may never fully understand it. But *you* will.

And that's more than enough.

Chapter 3 Summary:

Redefining Success and Slowing Down was about breaking away from the idea that more equals better. We explored how:

- Constant productivity is a myth that leads to burnout.
- Shifting to a balanced mindset reclaims our energy.
- Rest is not laziness — it's necessary.
- Slow living isn't old-fashioned; it's revolutionary.
- Saying "no" is a form of self-respect, not selfishness.
- A good life isn't about appearances — it's about alignment.

Peace isn't found at the finish line. It's found in the pauses — and in the life you create from your truest self.

Chapter 4: Reconnecting With Your Body

Section 1: Where Stress Hides in Your Muscles and Gut

Take a moment and check in with yourself — how does your body feel right now?

Is your jaw tight? Shoulders raised toward your ears? A persistent flutter in your stomach? Maybe you're clenching your fists without realizing it, or your breath has been shallow for hours. These small cues might seem insignificant, but they're actually major clues: your body has been whispering to you. The question is, have you been listening?

Welcome to Chapter 4 — where we shift focus from our thoughts to the vessel that carries them: our bodies.

In the past three chapters, we explored the cultural, technological, and lifestyle contributors to chronic anxiety. We looked at how external pressures shape our internal chaos. But there's one element we haven't yet explored deeply: how this anxiety settles physically inside us. Because anxiety isn't just a mental storm — it's a physical experience too.

And more often than not, our bodies know we're anxious before our minds do.

The Body's Anxiety Blueprint

The connection between body and mind is not a vague spiritual idea; it's biology. Every time you feel anxious, your brain signals your body that something is wrong. It sends cortisol and adrenaline pumping through your system —

preparing you to run or fight. This might be helpful if you're facing a tiger. But when your stressor is a missed deadline, a pile of bills, or an argument left unresolved, the body doesn't know the difference.

So what happens? The response gets stuck. Your muscles tense. Your digestive system slows down. Your heart races. Your breathing becomes shallow. Your palms sweat. And all of this becomes your new default mode.

In other words, your body is living as if it's under constant threat.

Where Stress Lives: Muscles, Gut, and More

Let's break it down. Where, specifically, does anxiety show up in the body?

1. The Jaw

Grinding teeth at night or clenching your jaw during the day? This is one of the most common physical manifestations of stress. The temporomandibular joint (TMJ) is often strained under chronic anxiety, leading to tension headaches and even ear pain.

2. The Shoulders and Neck

You might say, "I carry the weight of the world on my shoulders." And guess what? Your body agrees. The trapezius and neck muscles are usually the first to tighten when you're under pressure. This constant contraction can cause stiffness, migraines, and upper back pain.

3. The Stomach and Gut

Have you ever had "butterflies" before a big moment? Or felt like you had a "knot" in your stomach during a difficult conversation? That's your gut-brain axis in action. Your digestive system is deeply connected to your mental state. Anxiety can cause nausea, bloating, indigestion, constipation, or diarrhea. In fact, IBS (Irritable Bowel Syndrome) is often closely tied to chronic stress.

4. The Chest and Heart

Shortness of breath? Tight chest? Racing heart? These are textbook signs of anxiety's impact. Your cardiovascular and respiratory systems are often hijacked when you're mentally overwhelmed, even if you're not aware of it.

5. The Hands and Feet

Cold or sweaty palms. Tingling fingers. Restless feet. These subtle signals are your body saying: "I'm ready to bolt." The fight-or-flight response reallocates blood flow to prepare for action — which can leave your extremities feeling strange.

6. Sleep Patterns

Your body doesn't forget. If you're always on alert, your sleep becomes shallow, interrupted, or delayed. You may not even feel rested after a full night's sleep because your body never got a chance to truly relax.

Listening to the Body: A Skill We Forgot

Somewhere along the line — between the busy schedules, the digital distractions, and the social performance — we stopped listening to our bodies. We became so used to the tension that it became normal.

We are taught to think through our problems, but rarely are we taught to feel through them.

Your body has its own language. It speaks in aches, in fatigue, in shortness of breath, in tightness. It begs for pauses and stretches and deep, intentional breaths. But we've learned to override its signals in favor of "pushing through."

If this resonates with you, you're not alone. Many people in our anxious generation have been disconnected from their bodies for years. Reconnection can feel strange at first — even uncomfortable. But it's essential.

How to Start Reconnecting With Your Body

So, what can you do?

You don't need to book a retreat or turn your life upside down. Here are some simple yet powerful ways to start tuning in again:

1. Body Scan Meditation

Lie down or sit comfortably. Close your eyes. Starting from your toes, slowly bring your attention to each part of your body, noticing any tension or sensation. No judgment — just awareness.

2. Daily Check-ins

Ask yourself, "How does my body feel today?" Do this at least once in the morning and once at night. Write it down if it helps.

3. Gentle Movement

Yoga, stretching, or even a short walk can work wonders. Move in a way that feels nurturing, not punishing.

4. Breathwork

Anxiety shortens our breath. Try inhaling for four counts, holding for four, exhaling for four, and pausing for four (box breathing). Do this for a minute and see how your body responds.

5. Release Tension Intentionally

Progressive muscle relaxation involves tensing and then releasing each muscle group from head to toe. It helps your body relearn what "relaxed" even feels like.

Your Body as an Ally, Not an Enemy

Here's the big takeaway: your body isn't working against you. It's trying to protect you.

When you feel pain, tightness, or unease — it's not punishment. It's communication.

Anxiety shows up physically because your body is loyal. It reacts even when you're too distracted to notice. That loyalty is a gift. And when we learn to treat our bodies not as machines to be pushed, but as partners to be cared for, healing begins.

You don't need to become a yoga expert or a mindfulness guru. You just need to start by paying attention. The calm you're searching for isn't just a mindset — it's a full-body experience.

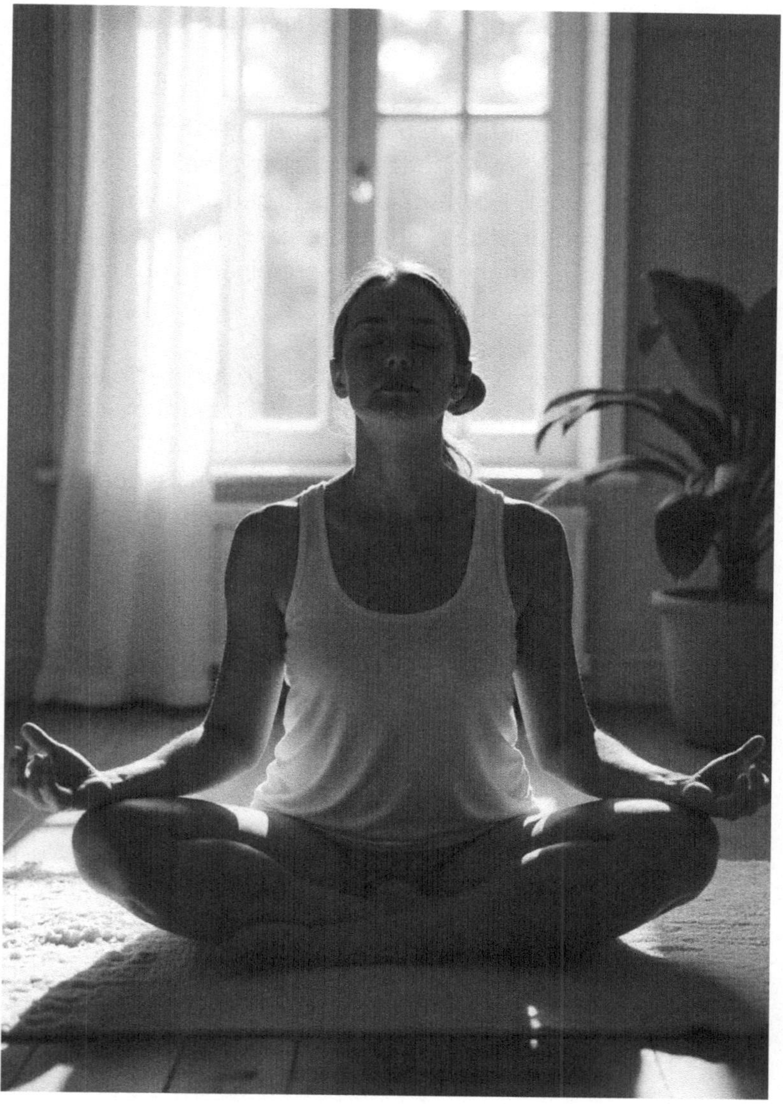

Section 2: Breath, Stillness, and the Nervous System Reset

Imagine this: you're sitting in traffic, running late for an important meeting. Your hands are gripping the steering wheel a little too tightly, your jaw is clenched, and your shoulders are scrunched up near your ears. Your heart beats a little faster, your thoughts begin to spiral, and you're barely breathing. Sound familiar?

That experience—tight muscles, shallow breath, racing heart—is your nervous system in fight-or-flight mode. It's how your body responds when it senses danger. But in today's world, "danger" often comes in the form of emails, deadlines, arguments, or traffic—not wild animals. And yet, our bodies still react the same way.

This is where breath and stillness come in. They are not just feel-good practices taught in yoga studios. They are biological tools. They are levers we can pull when our nervous system feels hijacked. They help signal to the brain, "You're safe now. You can calm down."

Let's unpack how breath and stillness can help us reclaim calm—not just in theory, but in real, grounded, everyday ways.

The Science of Breath

Breath is the one function in your body that is both automatic and under your control. You don't need to think to breathe—but you can choose how to breathe. And that choice changes everything.

When you take a slow, deep breath, something magical (and scientific) happens. Your vagus nerve, which runs from your brainstem down to your gut, gets activated. This nerve is a key part of your parasympathetic nervous system—the "rest and digest" mode. When it's triggered, your heart rate slows down, digestion resumes, your muscles relax, and your body exits survival mode.

On the flip side, shallow, fast breathing keeps you locked in the sympathetic nervous system—"fight or flight." It tells your body you're in danger, even when you're not.

Try This Now: Take a slow, deep breath in for a count of four. Hold it gently for a count of four. Exhale slowly for a count of six. Repeat three times.

Notice any change in how you feel. Even a subtle shift matters. That's your nervous system responding. That's power in your pocket.

Stillness Is Not Inactivity

Stillness isn't about doing nothing. It's about intentional pause. It's the act of *being* instead of constantly *doing*. And in a world that glorifies hustle, stillness feels almost rebellious.

When you sit quietly, even for just five minutes, you give your brain a chance to stop reacting and start regulating. You allow your body to shift out of emergency mode and return to balance.

Stillness gives us space to notice: "Oh, I didn't realize my stomach was tense," or "Wow, I've been clenching my fists." That awareness is the beginning of regulation.

Stillness can look like:

- Sitting on your porch and watching the trees move
- Closing your eyes during a lunch break and breathing
- Pausing before replying to a stressful email
- Lying on the floor with your hand on your chest

Stillness doesn't have to mean silence or meditation. It just means choosing a moment of non-reaction.

The Power of the Pause

In every stressful moment, there's a tiny pause—a sliver of space between stimulus and response. Most of us miss it because we're moving too fast. But when we learn to *live in that pause*, we start to make different choices. Calmer choices.

Let's say you get a critical text message. Your chest tightens. Your fingers twitch, ready to respond. But what if you paused for 10 seconds? Took one slow breath. Re-centered. Then responded.

That tiny breath-fueled pause could be the difference between a regret-filled reply and a calm boundary. That pause is emotional self-defense. It's your nervous system's version of putting on armor—without aggression.

Breathwork Practices You Can Try

You don't need to attend a fancy retreat or become a monk to use breath as medicine. You just need awareness and consistency.

Here are three simple techniques:

1. **Box Breathing**

- Inhale for 4 counts
- Hold for 4 counts
- Exhale for 4 counts
- Hold for 4 counts
- Repeat for 4 rounds

Used by Navy SEALs and therapists alike, this method brings balance and calm.

2. **4-7-8 Breath**

- Inhale for 4
- Hold for 7
- Exhale for 8
- Repeat 3-4 times

Great for falling asleep or easing anxiety.

3. **Diaphragmatic Breathing** (Belly Breathing)

- Place one hand on your chest, one on your belly
- Inhale deeply so your belly rises, chest remains still
- Exhale fully, feeling belly lower

This retrains your body to breathe deeply and fully.

Why This Works Across Cultures

Whether you're in bustling New York or a quiet village in Ghana, the biology is the same. Your nervous system speaks one language—safety. And breath is its translator.

That's why people in every culture have breath-centered practices:

- **India:** Pranayama in yoga
- **Japan:** Zen meditation
- **Africa:** Rhythmic drumming and communal chanting (breath syncing)
- **Middle East:** Sufi breathing techniques

Breath connects us globally. It's the thread between mindfulness in the East and stress-reduction science in the West.

Everyday Moments to Practice

You don't need to add breathwork to your to-do list. Instead, *weave it into what you're already doing.*

- Waiting in line? Breathe.
- Stuck in traffic? Breathe.
- Brushing your teeth? Breathe.
- Before a meeting? Breathe.
- After bad news? Pause, then breathe.

These micro-moments add up. They teach your nervous system that calm is always available, even in chaos.

Listening to Your Body with Compassion

Sometimes, stillness and breath can feel like too much—especially if you've spent years avoiding your body's signals. If emotions flood in, or tension surfaces, be kind. Don't judge. Just notice.

Imagine your body like a child who's been trying to get your attention. It's not trying to sabotage you. It's trying to say: "Hey, I need help." And with breath and stillness, you're finally listening.

A Tiny Shift, A Huge Impact

You don't need to become a meditation master overnight. Just start with one intentional breath. One pause. One silent moment. That's where change begins—not with grand gestures, but with gentle shifts.

Because the truth is: *Your breath is always with you.* It's your anchor, your reset button, your quiet superpower.

And every time you use it, you take one more step toward reclaiming calm—not just in your mind, but in your body too.

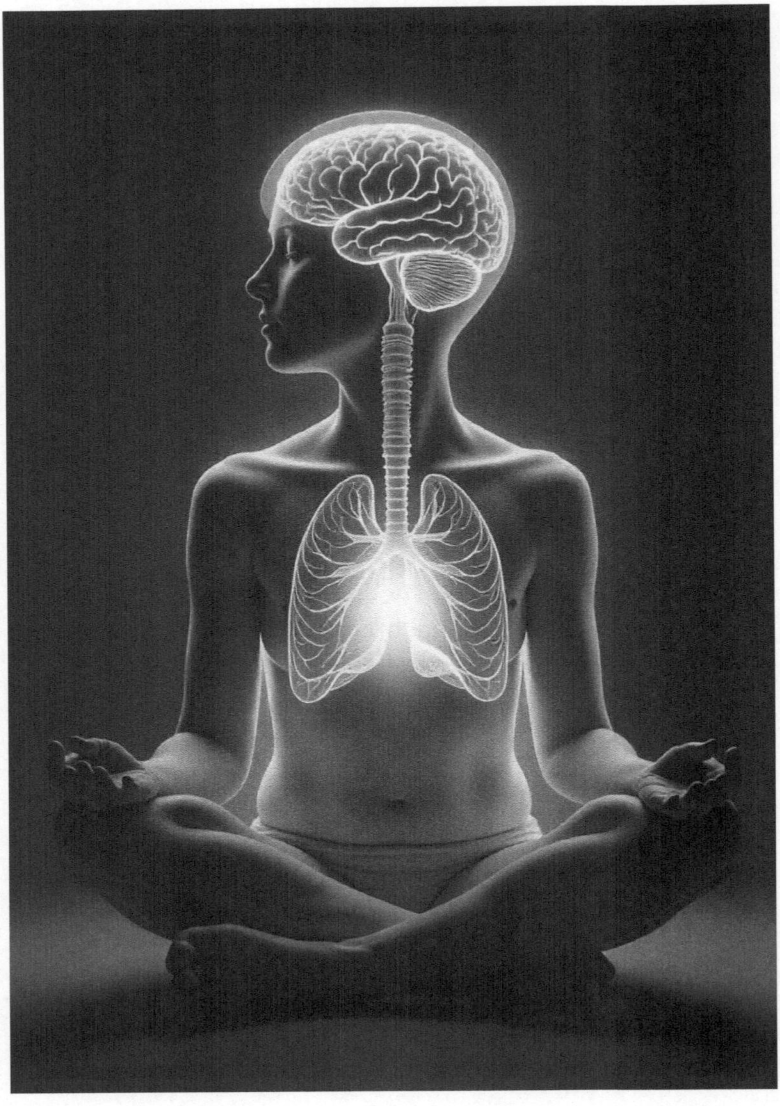

Section 3: Movement as Medicine (Without a Gym)

In a world obsessed with fitness culture, it's easy to think that movement only counts when it involves a gym membership, sweat-drenched gear, or an expensive tracking device. But movement is more than just burning calories or chasing a fitness goal — it's a powerful, underappreciated medicine for the anxious mind and tense body.

And here's the truth: healing movement isn't reserved for the fit, the flexible, or the Instagram-famous. You don't need to lift weights or run marathons to feel the incredible physical and emotional relief that comes with moving your body. In fact, sometimes the simplest movements — a walk, a stretch, a dance in your kitchen — can do more for your mental health than an hour of cardio ever could.

Why Movement Matters for Anxiety

We've already explored how stress and anxiety aren't just in our heads — they show up in our shoulders, our guts, our jaws, and our posture. Movement is one of the fastest ways to tell the nervous system: "You're safe."

When we move, we breathe deeper. Our blood flows better. Tense muscles relax. Movement also triggers the release of endorphins — our body's natural painkillers and mood boosters — as well as serotonin and dopamine, which are crucial to feelings of well-being.

But there's more. Movement helps regulate the autonomic nervous system (the same system responsible for fight-or-flight responses), lowers cortisol levels, and even helps recalibrate our circadian rhythm for better sleep.

Rethinking "Exercise"

One of the biggest mindset shifts we can embrace is redefining what movement means. In the context of healing anxiety, movement is not punishment. It's not about weight loss, perfect form, or progress photos. It's about connection — reconnecting with your breath, your body, and the present moment.

So let's ditch the toxic "no pain, no gain" narrative. What if we replaced it with: "No pressure, just presence"?

Small, Consistent Movements That Make a Big Impact

You don't need fancy equipment or a big block of time. You just need a few moments and a little willingness to be with your body. Here are some powerful, gym-free movements that are gentle on the body but big on mental wellness:

1. Walking

Walking is one of the most underrated therapeutic tools we have. It's free, accessible, and research shows it can significantly reduce symptoms of anxiety and depression. Walking in nature — also known as "green exercise" — adds another layer of calm.

Start small: a 10-minute stroll after meals, walking while listening to soothing music or an uplifting podcast, or even pacing in your living room while brainstorming or decompressing from the day.

2. Stretching and Mobility Flows

Stretching isn't just for athletes. Gentle stretching, particularly when done slowly and mindfully, helps release stored tension in the hips, shoulders, and back — the areas where we often store emotional stress.

You don't need to do a full yoga session. Even a five-minute morning stretch routine can reset your nervous system.

Try This:

- Neck rolls
- Shoulder shrugs
- Seated forward bends
- Child's pose
- Gentle spinal twists

3. Dance

You don't have to be a trained dancer to move to music. Dancing freely — in your bedroom, kitchen, or backyard — is an emotional release. Movement with music engages the emotional and creative parts of the brain and can uplift your mood in minutes.

Put on a song you love and let your body lead. No choreography needed.

4. Grounding Movement

Try barefoot movement like gentle yoga or tai chi in your home or yard. Grounding (or "earthing") — direct contact with the ground — can reduce inflammation, balance cortisol, and promote emotional regulation.

Combine grounding with deep breathing for maximum effect.

5. Desk and Chair Movement

If you're spending most of your day at a desk, micro-movements matter. Every hour, stand up, stretch, twist your spine, roll your shoulders. Even doing leg lifts or shoulder rolls while seated can prevent the kind of muscle tightening that contributes to anxiety.

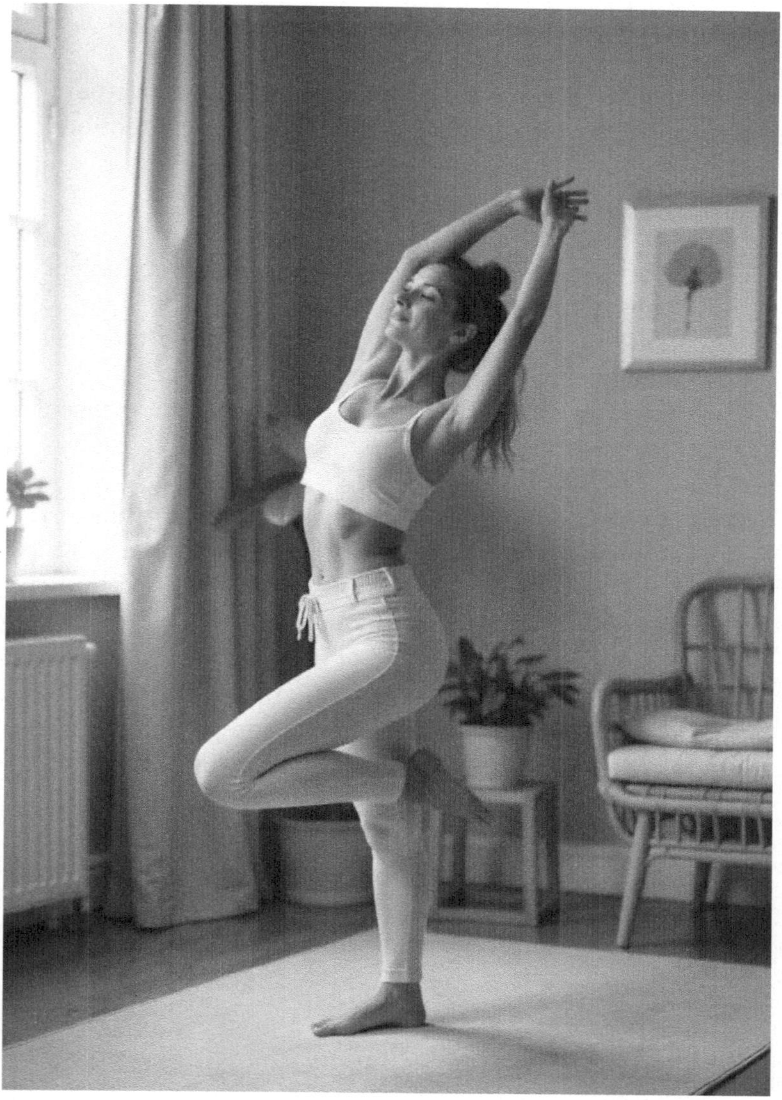

Creating a Movement Ritual

We thrive on rhythm. Creating a daily or weekly movement ritual doesn't have to be rigid — but it should be intentional.

Here are a few ideas:

- **Morning movement:** 5-10 minutes of stretching or walking to set the tone.
- **Midday reset:** Step outside for a breath of fresh air and a short walk.
- **Evening unwind:** Gentle yoga or dance to release the day's tension.

Keep it joyful. Keep it light. Your movement doesn't have to "achieve" anything. Its value lies in how it makes you feel.

Listening to Your Body, Not Pushing It

One of the reasons people give up on exercise routines is because they were built around shame, comparison, or over-exertion. When your body is already carrying the weight of stress and anxiety, the last thing it needs is more pressure.

Instead, move from a place of kindness. If your body says rest, honor that. If it craves movement, give it gently. Over time, this respectful approach builds trust between you and your body.

Mindful Movement Mantra:

"I move to listen. I move to heal. I move because I matter."

Movement as a Gateway to Stillness

Interestingly, many people find that it's movement — not stillness — that eventually leads them to moments of clarity and peace. After a walk or a gentle stretch, your nervous system is calmer, your breath is deeper, your mind is quieter.

This is why movement can be such a powerful companion to other healing practices like meditation or journaling. It gets us out of the noise in our heads and into the safety of our bodies.

A Universal Tool for a Global Reader

Wherever you are in the world — a high-rise in Tokyo, a rural village in Kenya, a suburban home in Canada — movement is available to you. You don't need perfect weather, a fitness background, or special equipment.

You just need a body that wants to be heard and honored. Movement is the language it speaks.

Section 4: Eating for Energy and Emotional Resilience

Food is not just fuel; it is information. Every bite you take sends messages to your brain and body about how to function, how to respond to stress, and how to heal. When we eat with intention, we give ourselves the tools to build resilience — not just physically, but emotionally and mentally. In this section, we explore how your plate can become a powerful foundation for calm, clarity, and connection.

The Gut-Brain Connection: A Two-Way Street

Have you ever felt butterflies in your stomach before a big event? Or lost your appetite during an anxious time? That's your gut-brain axis at work. The gut and brain are constantly communicating through the vagus nerve, sending chemical signals that impact mood, digestion, and stress response.

Roughly 90% of the body's serotonin (the "feel good" hormone) is produced in the gut. A healthy digestive system supports the production of neurotransmitters that regulate mood and energy. When the gut is imbalanced — inflamed, overwhelmed, or undernourished — it can lead to symptoms like fatigue, irritability, brain fog, and increased anxiety.

Mood-Food: What to Eat (and Why It Matters)

Eating for emotional resilience means choosing foods that nourish both your body and mind. Here are the key categories to focus on:

1. Complex Carbohydrates

Whole grains like oats, brown rice, and quinoa provide steady energy and support serotonin production. Unlike refined sugars that spike and crash your blood sugar, complex carbs fuel your brain in a balanced way.

2. Healthy Fats

Omega-3 fatty acids, found in fatty fish (like salmon and sardines), flaxseeds, walnuts, and chia seeds, are crucial for brain health. Studies have shown that omega-3s can reduce symptoms of anxiety and depression.

3. Protein-Rich Foods

Proteins are made up of amino acids, which are the building blocks of neurotransmitters. Lean meats, legumes, eggs, and dairy support alertness, focus, and a stable mood.

4. Fiber and Prebiotics

Vegetables, fruits, and legumes are rich in fiber and prebiotics that feed your gut microbiome. A diverse gut flora boosts your immune system and reduces inflammation, which is linked to chronic stress.

5. Probiotic Foods

Fermented foods like yogurt, kefir, sauerkraut, kimchi, and kombucha contain beneficial bacteria that directly support gut health and mood regulation.

6. Hydrating Foods and Water

Even mild dehydration can increase stress levels and impair cognitive performance. Include water-dense foods like cucumbers, oranges, watermelon, and herbal teas in your daily intake.

What to Reduce: Foods That Drain Your Calm

Just as some foods build your resilience, others deplete it.

- **Excess Sugar:** Causes blood sugar spikes, followed by crashes that trigger irritability and anxiety.
- **Caffeine Overload:** A small amount can be helpful, but too much stimulates the nervous system and worsens anxiety.
- **Highly Processed Foods:** Packaged snacks, fast food, and trans fats increase inflammation and disrupt the gut-brain axis.
- **Alcohol:** Initially sedating, alcohol disrupts sleep, blood sugar, and serotonin balance over time.

These aren’t foods you need to cut out entirely, but being mindful of their effects can help you make better choices.

Eating Patterns That Support Peace

It's not just *what* you eat, but *how* you eat that matters. Mindful eating is a practice that can transform your relationship with food:

- **Slow Down:** Eating slowly gives your digestive system time to activate and your mind time to process satiety.
- **Eat Without Screens:** Multitasking with social media or TV increases stress and disconnects you from your body’s cues.
- **Check in Emotionally:** Before eating, ask yourself: Am I hungry, or am I bored, anxious, or sad?
- **Create Rituals:** Light a candle, say a word of gratitude, and eat at a table instead of your desk. These small habits ground your nervous system.

Cultural Wisdom and Emotional Eating

Many traditional cuisines around the world have built-in patterns that promote calm and connection:

- **Mediterranean Diet:** Rich in olive oil, fish, vegetables, legumes, and social mealtime traditions.
- **Japanese Meals:** Include fermented foods like miso and natto, portion control, and balanced flavors.
- **Indian Ayurveda:** Encourages mindful eating, seasonal foods, and digestion-supportive spices like turmeric and cumin.

Reclaiming your cultural food roots (or respectfully exploring others) can bring emotional grounding and pleasure to your meals.

When Food Becomes a Coping Mechanism

In stressful times, food can become a source of control or comfort. Emotional eating is natural, but when it becomes habitual, it may block you from fully feeling or processing your emotions.

Instead of judging yourself for emotional eating, try using it as a signal. What are you really hungry for? Connection, rest, creativity, love?

Shifting from punishment ("I shouldn't have eaten that") to curiosity ("What was I feeling before I reached for that?") creates space for change without shame.

Practical Tips for Every Budget and Lifestyle

Eating well doesn't have to be expensive or complicated. Here's how to make it accessible:

- **Batch Cooking:** Prepare meals in advance so you're less likely to grab processed foods in a rush.
- **Smart Snacking:** Keep nuts, fruits, and boiled eggs on hand instead of sugary snacks.
- **One Upgrade at a Time:** Swap white rice for brown, soda for herbal tea, or chips for carrot sticks.
- **Community Sharing:** Cook with friends, trade meals, or start a healthy recipe swap.

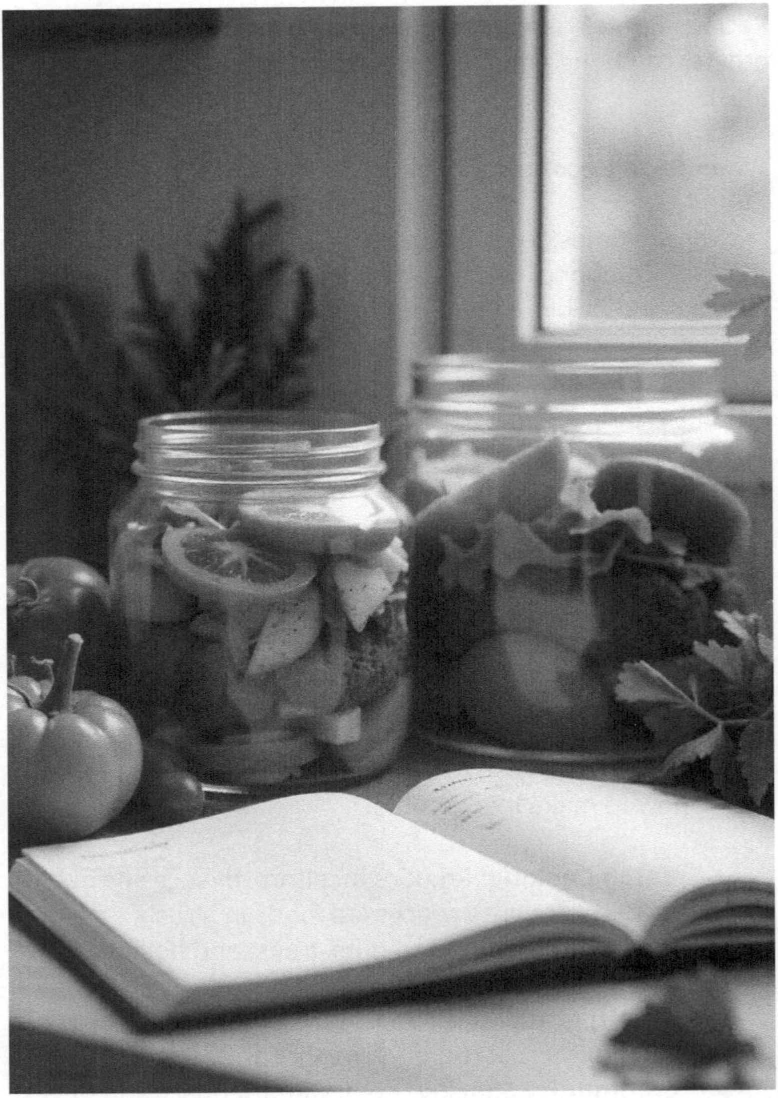

Emotional Resilience Starts with Nourishment

Every cell in your body relies on nutrients to function. When we provide our bodies with consistent, loving nourishment, we lay the groundwork for emotional regulation, mental clarity, and grounded energy.

Eating isn't just about avoiding illness or maintaining weight. It's about nurturing your nervous system, honoring your needs, and choosing peace every time you sit down to a plate.

Your next meal isn't just food. It's an invitation to return to yourself.

Section 5: Sleep: Your Free and Forgotten Therapy

In the race of daily responsibilities, sleep has quietly slipped from our list of priorities. It's now common, almost a badge of honor, to declare how little sleep we've had, equating exhaustion with commitment, and rest with weakness. But here's the truth: sleep isn't laziness. It's not a luxury. It's a built-in, no-cost, deeply restorative therapy. And many of us are sleep-deprived in ways we don't even recognize.

Sleep is where your body resets, your mind files memories, and your emotions are gently sorted out. If you've ever woken up more tired than when you went to bed, or experienced brain fog that coffee can't fix, this section is for you.

The Science Behind Sleep and Stress Relief

Sleep plays a central role in regulating the nervous system. When we're asleep—particularly during deep, non-REM and REM stages—our bodies process cortisol levels, manage emotional memory, and activate healing responses. Lack of sufficient sleep leads to elevated stress hormones, weakened immune response, increased inflammation, and impaired decision-making. It's like trying to run on a phone stuck at 10% battery—anxious, glitchy, and constantly crashing.

Studies show that even moderate sleep deprivation (just getting six hours instead of seven to nine) can lead to increased irritability, reduced emotional resilience, and higher perceived stress. In short: the less you sleep, the more everything feels like a crisis.

Modern Life and the Sleep Crisis

Several factors contribute to the global sleep crisis:

- **Screen Time:** Blue light from phones and laptops suppresses melatonin, the hormone responsible for sleep.
- **Late-night stimulation:** Scrolling social media, watching intense shows, or checking work emails all prime the brain for alertness—not sleep.
- **Irregular schedules:** Shift work, late-night productivity habits, and inconsistent sleep/wake times confuse our internal circadian rhythm.
- **Caffeine dependence:** Many drink coffee late into the afternoon to fight fatigue, which disrupts natural sleep patterns.

We treat sleep like a backup plan rather than a cornerstone of health.

Mini Reflection Exercise: Ask yourself:

- Do I view sleep as essential, or something I fit in if there's time?

- When was the last time I felt truly rested?
- Am I more anxious, reactive, or scattered when I sleep poorly?

Awareness is the first step. Without guilt, just notice what's true for you.

Sleep and Emotional Recovery

Ever notice how problems feel more manageable after a good night's rest? That's not your imagination. During sleep, particularly in the REM phase, the brain replays and reprocesses emotional events. This helps soften their sting and integrate them more peacefully into our memory banks.

Sleep acts like a therapist—processing heartbreak, anxiety, insecurity, and stress while we rest. But when we rob ourselves of deep sleep, we carry yesterday's emotional baggage into today, heavier and more tangled.

Building a Sleep Ritual (Not Just a Routine)

A sleep ritual isn't about a strict schedule; it's about sending signals to your body that rest is coming. It's a transition from the outer world to your inner sanctuary.

Here are some intentional, calming steps to try:

- **Dim the lights** an hour before bed to mimic sunset.
- **Limit screens** or use blue light filters after 8 pm.
- **Sip herbal tea** like chamomile, lemon balm, or lavender.
- **Stretch gently** or do calming breathwork for 5 minutes.
- **Journal** your thoughts to clear mental clutter.

- **Use essential oils** like lavender, frankincense, or cedarwood.
- **Play soft ambient music** or sleep sounds (rain, waves, wind).

Rituals are powerful because they create consistency and safety—a deep signal to your nervous system that it's okay to let go.

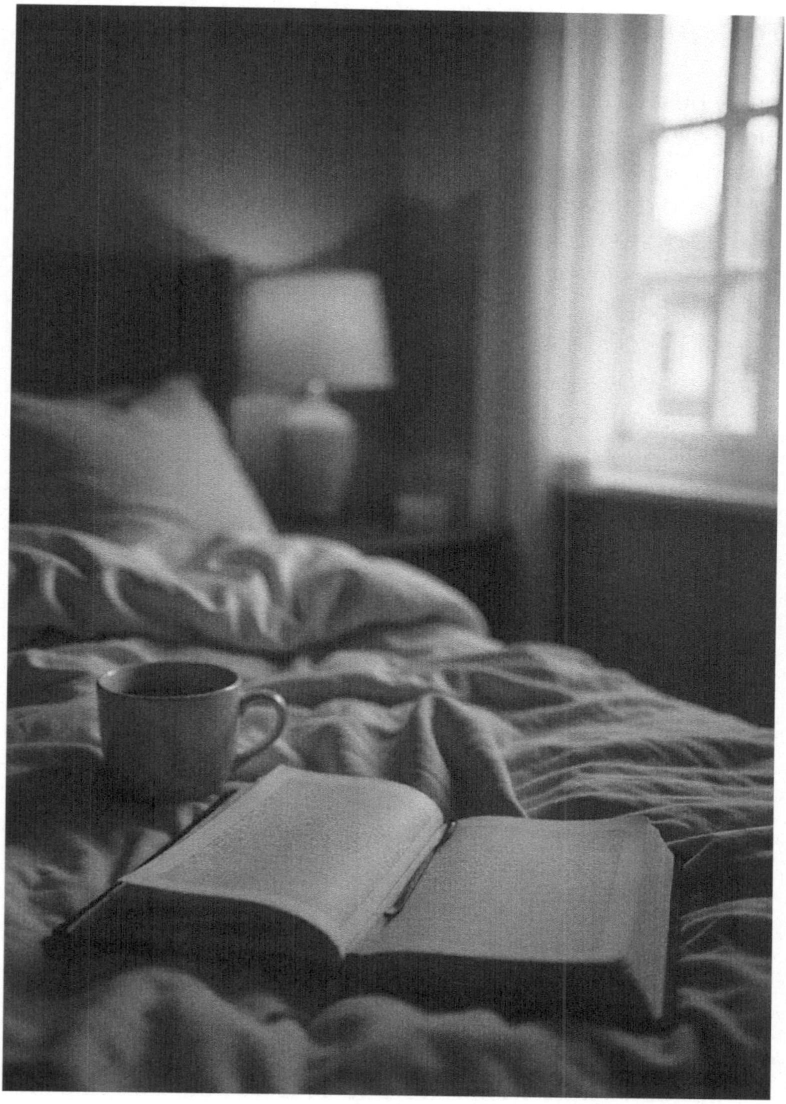

The Myth of Catching Up on Sleep

Many believe they can sleep five hours on weekdays and binge-sleep on weekends to recover. Unfortunately, sleep doesn't work like a savings account. You can't withdraw all week and deposit back in on Saturday. Research shows that even short-term sleep debt impairs cognition, metabolism, and mood, and the brain rarely 'recovers' in full from chronic deprivation.

Consistency is more important than quantity. It's better to get 7 hours consistently than swing between 4 and 10 unpredictably.

What Quality Sleep Feels Like

Good sleep isn't just the number of hours—it's the depth and consistency. Signs of quality sleep include:

- Falling asleep within 15–20 minutes
- Staying asleep through the night (or waking briefly and returning easily)
- Waking up without an alarm (eventually)
- Feeling alert and focused during the day

If these feel far from your reality, you're not alone—but there is hope.

Troubleshooting Common Sleep Issues

1. **Can't fall asleep:** Avoid screens an hour before bed. Try journaling, herbal supplements like magnesium glycinate, or meditative breathing.
2. **Waking at 3 a.m.:** This is often linked to cortisol spikes. Avoid sugar and caffeine late in the day and

consider gentle blood sugar balancing snacks like almonds or bananas before bed.

3. **Restless mind:** Try a guided body scan meditation or keep a 'worry notebook' to release racing thoughts.

Pro Tip: Instead of forcing sleep, focus on creating a restful environment and mindset. Even lying in bed calmly with closed eyes helps regulate the nervous system.

The Sleep-Anxiety Spiral

Poor sleep worsens anxiety. Anxiety disrupts sleep. It's a vicious cycle. Breaking it starts with one step: prioritize sleep as the foundation for your healing, not the last resort.

Sleep helps recalibrate your ability to handle stress. It boosts emotional regulation, increases resilience, and restores physical energy so you can meet life with more ease and clarity.

Quote to Reflect On: "Your future depends on your dreams, so go to sleep." – Mesut Barazany

Global Wisdom on Rest

Across cultures, rest has been revered—not resisted. In Spain, siestas are still part of traditional life. In Japan, inemuri (sleeping on the job) shows you're hardworking. In India, afternoon rest after a big lunch is common in many households. But in much of the modern West, rest has been falsely equated with laziness.

Let's reclaim the sacred value of sleep and rest, globally and personally.

Gentle Goals for Better Sleep

Start with what feels doable. A few options:

- Set a fixed bedtime and wake-up time for just 5 nights.
- Turn off screens 30 minutes before bed.
- Create a wind-down playlist.
- Try 4-7-8 breathing in bed: inhale for 4 seconds, hold for 7, exhale for 8.

Don't aim for perfection. Aim for peace.

Final Thought

If anxiety and modern overwhelm are taking a toll on your body, sleep is not optional—it's essential. This free, restorative tool is within reach, but it starts with giving it the value it deserves. Let's stop glorifying burnout and start honoring rest.

Section 6: Creating a Rhythm That Soothes You Daily

We live in a world that moves quickly. Emails, text messages, and push notifications never sleep. Meals are rushed. Even leisure is scheduled down to the minute. In all this chaos, our nervous system—the delicate wiring that connects our thoughts to our physical bodies—is silently overwhelmed. Chapter 4 has walked us through the profound truth that anxiety isn't only in the mind, but also in the body. We've explored how stress nests in our muscles, the healing power of stillness and breath, the medicine of movement, the connection between food and emotions, and the undervalued gift of sleep. Now we arrive at an essential piece: creating a daily rhythm that acts as both anchor and balm.

A rhythm is not the same as a rigid routine. Routines are often about productivity; rhythms are about peace. Routines can become a checklist; rhythms flow. Establishing a rhythm that supports your mental and physical well-being is one of the kindest things you can do for yourself.

Why Rhythms Matter to Your Nervous System

Imagine your nervous system as a musical instrument. If it's constantly overstimulated with discordant noise, it can't play its true melody. But when it is gently tuned with moments of calm, care, and predictability, it resonates with clarity. Daily rhythms offer predictability. Predictability creates safety. Safety reduces anxiety.

Many of us unknowingly live in what scientists call a "sympathetic dominant state," or the "fight or flight" mode. It means your body is constantly prepared for danger, even if there is no threat in front of you. This might show up as irritability, shallow breathing, clenched jaws, or insomnia. Rhythms help the body shift into its parasympathetic mode—the rest-and-digest state where healing happens.

Morning: Set the Tone for the Day

Your morning rhythm doesn't have to start at 5:00 a.m. or include a ten-step productivity checklist. It simply needs to nourish you before the world rushes in.

Here are gentle practices to include:

- **No phone for the first 30 minutes:** Let your nervous system wake up naturally before feeding it notifications or news.

- **Hydrate and move:** A glass of water and a few stretches signal to your body that it's safe and ready.
- **Breath check:** Start with three deep breaths to reconnect with your body. Inhale peace, exhale tension.
- **Intention setting:** Ask yourself, "What do I need today?" and listen without judgment.

Even five minutes of mindfulness in the morning can help center your day.

Midday: A Sacred Pause

In a culture that glorifies constant motion, taking a break can feel like rebellion. But midday pauses are not a luxury; they are necessary.

Create micro-rhythms throughout your day:

- **Eat without a screen:** Focus on your food. Chew slowly. Let it be a moment of nourishment.
- **Step outside:** Even five minutes of fresh air and natural light can reset your mood and focus.
- **Body scan:** Briefly check your shoulders, jaw, and breath. Are you holding tension?
- **Gratitude moment:** Name one thing going well, no matter how small.

These short pauses reduce cortisol levels and bring your nervous system back to baseline.

Evening: Transition With Intention

The evening is your chance to invite closure. Without transition rituals, many of us bring the chaos of the day into our sleep.

Here are ways to craft an evening rhythm:

- **Digital sunset:** One hour before bed, step away from screens.
- **Low lights and calming scents:** Signal to your body that it's time to slow down.
- **Light stretching or slow walk:** Help release tension built up throughout the day.
- **Reflective journaling:** What did you feel today? What are you proud of? What can you release?
- **Prayer or quiet meditation:** Center yourself before rest.

This is not about perfection. It's about compassion.

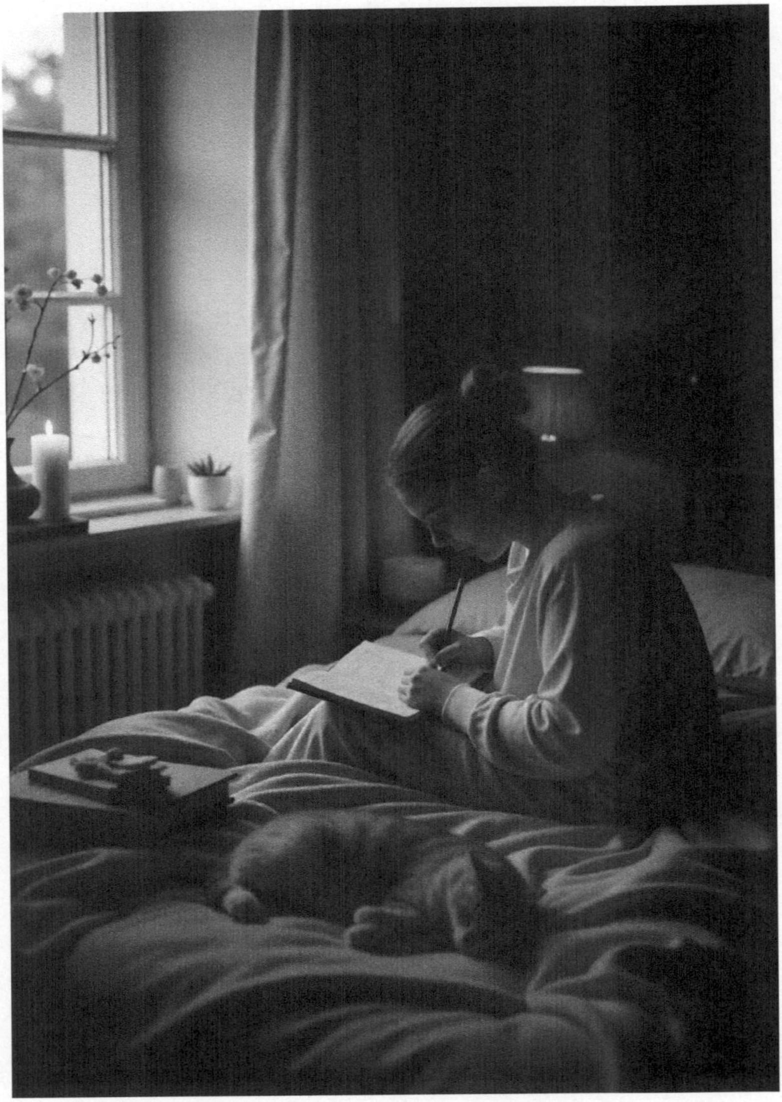

Weekly and Monthly Rhythms

While daily rhythms soothe our nervous system, zooming out to look at weekly and monthly patterns helps us stay grounded long-term.

- **Weekly check-in:** Every Sunday or a quiet day, ask: What do I need more of? Less of?
- **Digital Sabbath:** Choose one day (or half a day) where you unplug.
- **Plan moments of joy:** Coffee with a friend, a walk in nature, a day with no agenda.
- **Cycle with your energy:** Some weeks may need more rest; some will ask for action. Listen.

These larger rhythms prevent burnout and nourish joy.

Compassion Over Control

When building rhythms, it can be tempting to overplan. But remember: rhythms are not punishments; they are practices of self-respect. If you miss a day, it's okay. Start again tomorrow.

Be flexible. Life happens. The key is not perfection, but presence. Ask yourself regularly, "What soothes me? What stirs me?" Adjust your rhythms accordingly.

For example:

- If you feel drained, perhaps your rhythm needs more stillness.
- If you feel anxious, maybe your rhythm lacks grounding.

Your rhythm is a conversation with your body. Keep listening.

The Peace of Predictability

Children thrive with predictable rhythms, and so do adults. When your body knows what to expect, it can relax. This is why cultures throughout history have embraced rituals—from morning prayers to mealtime blessings.

Rituals rooted in rhythm:

- Lighting a candle every evening to signal rest
- Playing the same song each morning while making tea
- Having one quiet hour every Sunday

These acts of predictability nourish the nervous system and create moments of sacred pause in a noisy world.

Designing Your Own Daily Rhythm

No two rhythms will look the same. Some people need more silence. Others thrive with music and movement. The goal isn't to copy someone else's template but to design your own.

Here are prompts to get started:

- What is one thing that calms me every time?
- When during the day do I feel most overwhelmed?
- How can I add small moments of peace there?
- What rhythm would feel loving to my future self?

Start small. A rhythm built with love grows stronger each day.

Chapter 4 Summary: Reconnecting With Your Body

Anxiety isn't just mental; it shows up in our bodies. From muscle tension and shallow breath to disrupted digestion and poor sleep, the nervous system speaks through physical symptoms. In this chapter, we explored how to tune back into our body with tools like conscious breathwork, gentle movement, nourishing food, sleep, and restorative daily rhythms. The invitation is simple but profound: make your body a place where calm is possible.

By listening to your body's needs and responding with compassion rather than criticism, you begin to heal. Rhythms are how we remember who we are—not machines, but living beings who need care, space, and grace. Each breath, stretch, bite, and pause is a chance to reconnect.

Chapter 5: Finding Mental Quiet in a Loud World

Section 1: What Mental Noise Really Is

You don't have to run away to a mountain to find peace — just quiet the noise inside.

Picture this: you're sitting in a quiet room, no one around, no phone buzzing, no emails popping up. Yet your mind is racing. Thoughts tumble over each other like clothes in a dryer: worries about tomorrow, that awkward thing you said last week, your to-do list, your body image, your bank account. It's like your brain has its own background music—only it's not soothing. That, right there, is mental noise.

Mental noise is the clutter of thoughts, distractions, and internal chatter that keeps us from being present. Unlike external noise (honking horns, shouting, alerts), this kind is invisible but deeply influential. It's the buzz in the background of your brain that stops you from feeling at peace, even in moments designed for rest. Understanding it is the first step toward reclaiming your mental space.

The Anatomy of Mental Noise

Mental noise doesn't come from nowhere. It has ingredients. Some are deeply rooted in our history, while others are shaped by our fast-paced, always-on culture.

Here are a few key sources:

1. **Overthinking and Rumination**: Replaying past conversations, predicting future disasters, or crafting the perfect comeback. It creates emotional static.

2. **Information Overload**: Thanks to the internet, we now consume the equivalent of 174 newspapers a day. Our brains are not built for this.
3. **Perfectionism**: Holding ourselves to impossibly high standards turns every small decision into a stressful one.
4. **People-Pleasing**: Mentally rehearsing how to say yes when you want to say no. Worrying about how others perceive you drains focus.
5. **Inner Critic**: That voice that whispers, "You're not enough."
6. **Unprocessed Emotions**: Suppressed feelings eventually become background noise, rising to the surface as irritability or anxiety.

This mental noise builds like plaque in the mind. Over time, it reduces clarity, increases stress, and makes us feel disconnected—even from ourselves.

How Mental Noise Feels (and Why We Ignore It)

Mental noise doesn't just affect our thoughts—it shapes how we live.

- You scroll endlessly not because you're bored, but because you're avoiding the discomfort of your own mind.
- You multitask all day yet feel like nothing got done.
- You lie in bed exhausted, but sleep won't come.

Still, we often ignore these signals. Why? Because noise has become normal. Culturally, busyness is praised. Silence is suspicious. If your mind isn't racing, are you even trying hard enough?

But here's the truth: peace isn't found in a productivity hack or a perfect morning routine. It starts with noticing the noise, then slowly turning down the volume.

Why This Matters Now More Than Ever

The modern world rewards noise:

- Social media thrives on outrage and distraction.
- Workplaces often value speed over depth.
- News cycles are driven by fear, not reflection.

If we don't consciously protect our mental space, the world will fill it for us.

Mental noise keeps us reactive, not reflective. It leads us to:

- Make impulsive decisions.
- Disconnect from our bodies.
- Lose joy in simple moments.

A loud mind makes it harder to hear your own intuition. To feel God, or love, or even basic satisfaction.

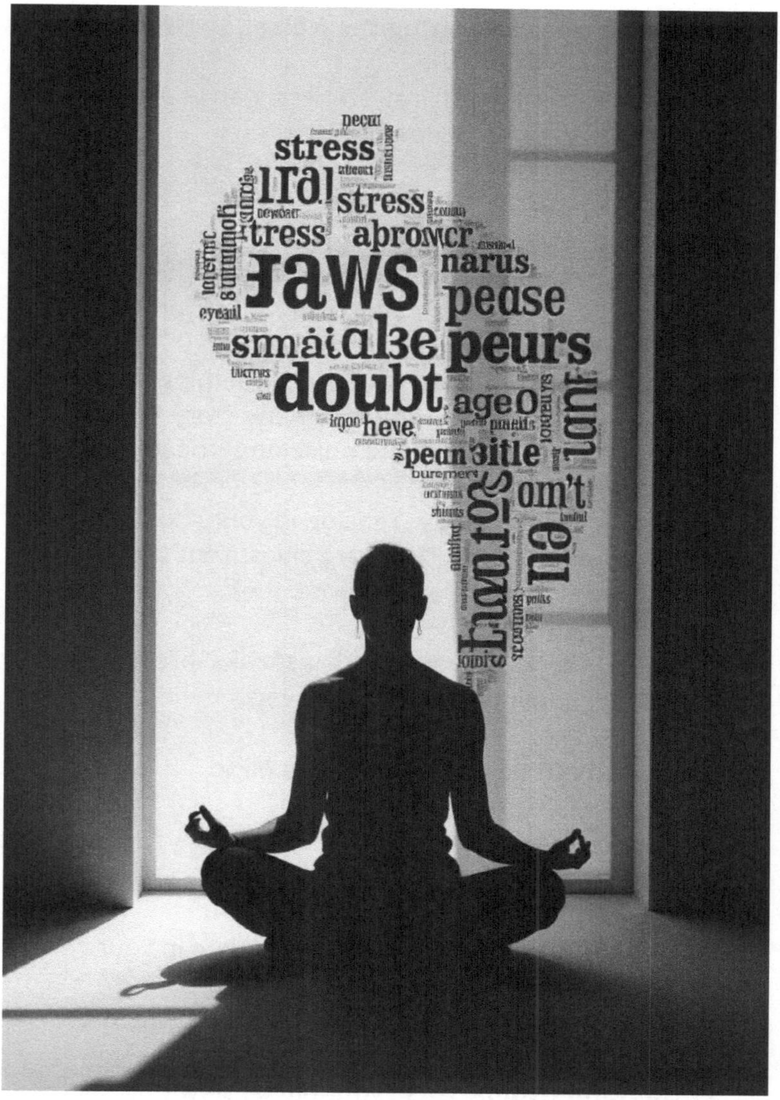
stress
stress
tress
narus
pease
peurs
doubt

Building Awareness: Spotting the Noise

The first step isn't silence. It's awareness. Can you spot mental noise in your daily life?

Try this:

- **Start a thought log**: For one day, every time you notice your mind spiraling or spinning, jot down the thought. Not to judge it. Just to see it.
- **Pause before reacting**: When something triggers you—an email, a comment, a news story—pause. Breathe. Ask: "What's the noise underneath this reaction?"
- **Listen to your body**: Tension in your shoulders? Stomach in knots? These are clues. Your body knows what your mind tries to ignore.

Mental noise isn't just in your head. It speaks through your posture, sleep, appetite, and energy levels.

Practical Steps to Begin Quieting the Mind

You don't need to become a monk or delete all your apps. But you can:

- **Schedule white space**: Put blank time in your calendar. Literally. Time for nothing.
- **Digital fast**: Choose a 2-hour window daily where you're offline. No exceptions.
- **Mindful rituals**: Wash your hands slowly. Drink tea with presence. Anchor your day with slowness.
- **Single-task**: Multitasking is a myth. Do one thing at a time, and do it with attention.

- **Talk to yourself kindly**: Catch your inner critic. Would you speak to a friend like that? Rewrite the message.

Mental Quiet Is a Practice, Not a Destination

Let's be honest. The noise won't disappear overnight. Some days it may even roar back louder than ever. But with practice, you start hearing the silence underneath.

The more you create space for stillness, the more mental quiet shows up uninvited—during a walk, in the shower, while watching a sunset.

This isn't about escaping the world. It's about being in it without being consumed by it.

You don't have to run away to a mountain to find peace. Just start by listening.

Section 2: The Power of Present Moment Awareness

We live in a world that constantly demands our attention. Phones buzz with alerts, deadlines loom like storm clouds, and even our leisure time is often spent multitasking. But amid this chaos, there is one ancient truth that modern science now echoes: peace can only be found in the present moment.

Present moment awareness is not about doing less, ignoring your responsibilities, or becoming someone new. It is about being where your feet are—fully, intentionally, and with compassion. It means quieting the mental noise not by escaping life but by arriving fully in it.

Why the Present Moment Is Powerful

Have you ever driven somewhere and realized you don't remember most of the journey? Or eaten a meal while scrolling your phone, only to forget what it tasted like? That's life without presence—life lived on autopilot.

Present moment awareness reclaims your experience. It allows you to witness your thoughts without being consumed by them, to feel emotions without judgment, and to make decisions from clarity instead of panic. It's not just calming—it's transformative.

When you're present, anxiety has less room to grow. Most of our stress is born from ruminating on the past or worrying about the future. But in the now, things are usually okay. Breathing in, you're alive. Breathing out, you have this moment. That is enough.

"You can't be both anxious and present. Choose presence, and anxiety begins to dissolve."

The Science of Being Here and Now

Neuroscientists have shown that present-moment practices like mindfulness and meditation can literally rewire your brain. They strengthen the prefrontal cortex (your rational, decision-making center) and quiet the amygdala (your fear and stress center). Regular practice can:

- Lower cortisol (the stress hormone)
- Improve focus and memory
- Reduce symptoms of anxiety and depression
- Increase emotional resilience

This isn't spiritual fluff. It's grounded in biology. When your brain learns to pause and notice the now, it spends less time catastrophizing, replaying old pain, or spinning worst-case scenarios.

What Does It Look Like to Be Present?

You don't need a meditation cushion, incense, or hours of silence. Present moment awareness can happen:

- While brushing your teeth — feeling the bristles, noticing the scent of the toothpaste.
- While walking — sensing the ground beneath your feet, the rhythm of your steps.
- While eating — savoring each bite, feeling gratitude for nourishment.
- While listening — being fully engaged, without thinking of your response.

Presence isn't a luxury; it's a skill. And like any skill, it grows with practice.

Barriers to Presence — and How to Break Through Them

Most of us resist presence without realizing it. Why? Because the present moment can feel uncomfortable. It may bring up sadness, boredom, guilt, or fear. That's why we run to distractions.

But the truth is, when you stay with discomfort long enough, it often softens. Your emotions, like waves, rise and fall. Presence teaches you to ride the wave instead of fighting it.

Common barriers include:

- **Overthinking**: Try labeling your thoughts—"planning," "judging," "remembering." This creates distance.
- **Distractions**: Turn off notifications. Create tech-free zones. Limit multitasking.
- **Restlessness**: Begin with small practices. Try one minute of presence instead of forcing an hour.

Presence is not about perfection. You will drift. That's okay. The practice is not in staying focused—it's in coming back. Again and again.

"The present moment is a doorway. Peace is what lies on the other side."

Practical Tools to Cultivate Present Moment Awareness

Here are a few methods to deepen your ability to be here, now:

1. The 5-4-3-2-1 Technique (Grounding)

Use your senses to anchor in the moment:

- 5 things you can see
- 4 things you can touch
- 3 things you can hear
- 2 things you can smell
- 1 thing you can taste

This brings your mind back into your body and your body into the now.

2. Box Breathing (Calming)

Inhale for 4 seconds, hold for 4 seconds, exhale for 4 seconds, hold for 4 seconds. Repeat. It activates your parasympathetic nervous system—your body's natural "rest and digest" mode.

3. Mindful Journaling (Reflective)

Ask yourself: *What am I feeling right now? What is happening in my body? What do I need in this moment?* Just a few sentences can create clarity.

4. Single-Tasking (Focused)

Choose one task. Do only that. Pour your attention into it. When distractions arise, gently return. You'll find joy in simple acts when they're done with presence.

5. Daily Mindfulness Ritual

Create a daily ritual—lighting a candle, stretching in the morning, washing your face slowly at night. Let these be moments of arrival.

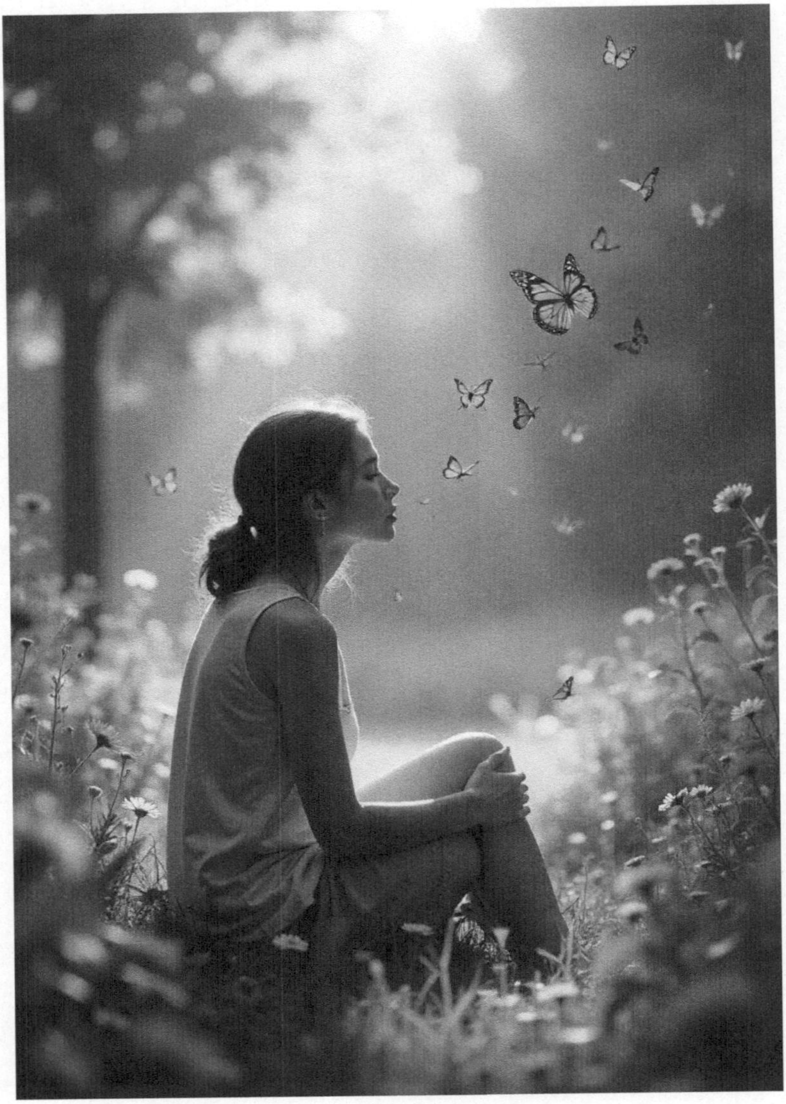

The Present Moment in Everyday Life

Presence can be your parenting style, your work ethic, your way of loving. It shows up when you listen without scrolling, when you eat without rushing, when you greet yourself with kindness in the mirror.

One mother shared that she began practicing presence during bedtime routines with her son. Instead of rushing through storytime, she slowed down. She noticed his laughter, the weight of his small hand in hers. "I thought I was too busy," she said. "But I was missing the most important parts of my life."

Presence won't erase your to-do list, but it will change how you move through it.

Common Misconceptions

"I don't have time to be present." You don't need more time. You just need to change how you use a few moments of it.

"Being present means ignoring problems." It's the opposite. Presence lets you face problems with a clear mind, not a chaotic one.

"I'm too anxious to be still." Stillness can be uncomfortable at first. But the more you practice, the more your nervous system learns it's safe to be calm.

What You'll Gain

- Clarity in decision-making
- A deeper connection to yourself and others
- Less emotional reactivity

- A renewed sense of peace
- Greater enjoyment of life's small moments

Presence isn't something you need to earn. It's available right now—in the breath you just took, in the page you're reading, in the quiet between your thoughts.

Section 3: Simple Grounding Practices for Real Life

In a world that pulls us in every direction at once—emails, to-do lists, the constant chatter of notifications and news updates—grounding can feel like a luxury. But it isn't. Grounding is not something reserved for yoga retreats or therapy offices. It's a deeply practical, everyday tool that helps us stay anchored in the present moment, especially when the storms of life feel too strong.

If you've ever felt like you're spinning mentally, like you're no longer in your own body or as if your thoughts are racing faster than your ability to catch up, grounding practices offer a reset button. In this section, we explore what grounding means, why it works, and how to incorporate it seamlessly into your daily life—no matter how busy or noisy the world around you might be.

What Is Grounding?

Grounding is the process of returning to the present moment by connecting to your body, your environment, or your senses. It's the opposite of dissociation, anxiety spirals, and future-focused worry. Grounding techniques act like a mental 'home base'—a place you can return to when your thoughts get loud and your emotions overwhelming.

Psychologists often use grounding in trauma therapy, but you don't need a diagnosis to benefit from it. Anyone dealing with stress, anxiety, or emotional overwhelm can use grounding as a form of daily mental hygiene.

Grounding is not about escapism. It's not about checking out, but rather about checking in. With yourself. With your breath. With the real world in front of you.

Why Grounding Works

Your brain is wired for survival, not peace. When your nervous system detects stress, it often defaults to fight, flight, or freeze. Grounding interrupts this cycle. It tells your brain: "I'm safe right now. I can slow down."

When you engage your senses in simple, repetitive activities, your brain shifts away from chaotic thinking and into the calm of the present. Grounding triggers your parasympathetic nervous system—the one responsible for rest and digestion—counteracting the effects of chronic stress and anxiety.

Real-Life Grounding Practices You Can Start Today

You don't need a meditation app or a candle-lit space to ground yourself. Here are practical, real-life techniques anyone can try:

1. The 5-4-3-2-1 Technique

This is one of the most popular and effective grounding tools for immediate relief.

- **5:** Acknowledge five things you can see.
- **4:** Acknowledge four things you can touch.

- **3:** Acknowledge three things you can hear.
- **2:** Acknowledge two things you can smell.
- **1:** Acknowledge one thing you can taste.

This technique pulls you out of your head and into your senses. It takes less than a minute and requires no equipment.

2. Barefoot Walking (Earthing)

Walking barefoot on natural surfaces like grass, sand, or soil connects your body with the Earth's electrical energy. Scientific studies suggest that earthing can reduce inflammation, improve sleep, and enhance mood.

Even five minutes of barefoot walking in your backyard or at a park can be incredibly restorative.

3. Breath + Touch

Place one hand over your heart and the other on your belly. Take slow, deep breaths. Feel the rise and fall. This physical connection to your breath and your body creates an instant feeling of safety and presence.

Do this before a meeting, after a tough conversation, or even while lying in bed.

4. Naming What's Real

When overwhelmed, say out loud:

- "I am sitting in a chair."
- "There is a plant on my desk."
- "My feet are on the ground."

This practice reinforces your connection to the present environment, breaking the cycle of rumination or panic.

5. Carry a Grounding Object

A small object in your pocket or bag—a smooth stone, a coin, a fabric swatch—can act as an anchor. Whenever anxiety spikes, hold it. Focus on its texture, temperature, and shape.

It sounds simple, but this tactile experience can bring your awareness back to the here and now.

6. Water Therapy

Run cold or warm water over your hands. Splash your face. Stand in the shower and pay attention to the sensations. Water has an incredibly soothing and cleansing quality—both physically and emotionally.

If you're near a natural body of water, even better. The sound and feel of water are powerful sensory tools.

7. Rhythmic Movement

Activities like walking, knitting, chopping vegetables, or even swaying gently can soothe the nervous system. Repetitive, rhythmic movement gives the mind a break and allows the body to find its own flow.

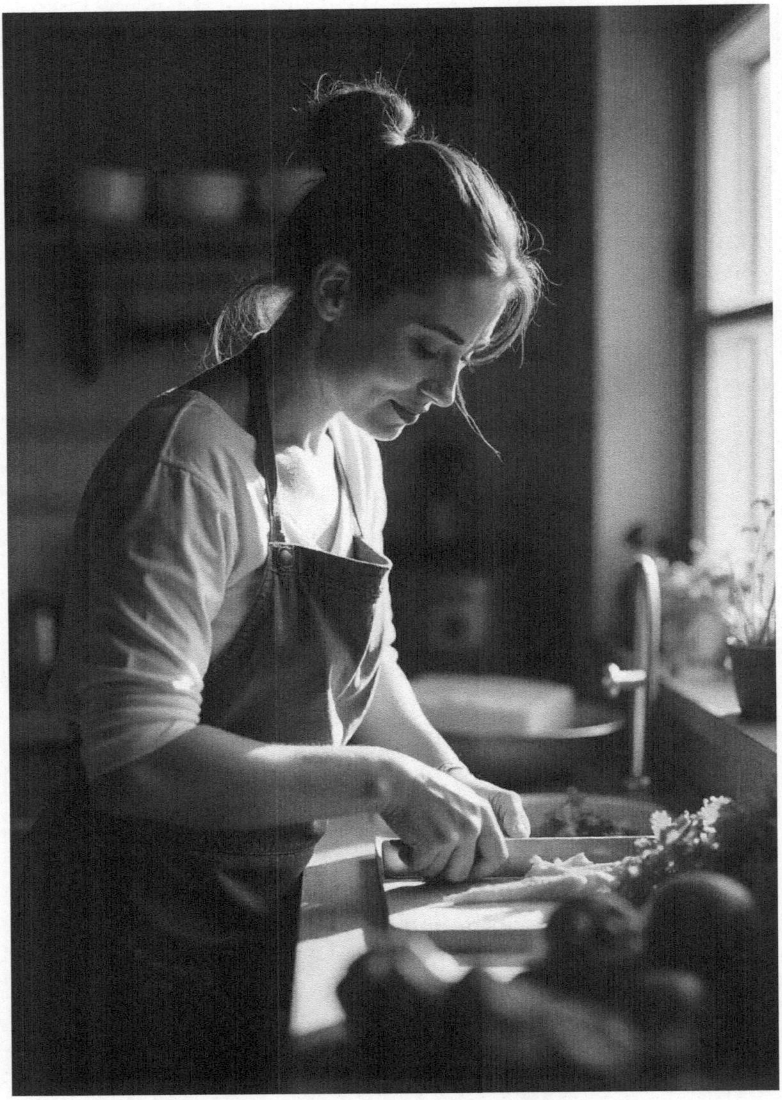

8. Anchor Your Day

Choose one simple grounding ritual to start and end your day. It could be a short breathing exercise, lighting a candle, journaling one line, or stretching for two minutes.

Consistency builds trust with yourself and signals your mind that you're safe and anchored.

Incorporating Grounding into a Busy Schedule

You may be thinking, "I don't have time for all of this."

Good news: grounding doesn't have to be long. In fact, shorter, more frequent moments are often more effective than one big session.

Try:

- Grounding for 60 seconds before you open your inbox.
- Doing 5 deep breaths in the bathroom stall before a meeting.
- Noticing the feeling of your steering wheel as you drive.
- Tuning in to your senses while washing dishes.

Grounding is not about doing more. It's about gently weaving awareness into what you already do.

Teaching Children (and Adults) to Ground

Kids, too, need grounding tools. When children are taught to connect with their bodies and environments, they grow up with emotional resilience.

Simple methods like breathing with a stuffed animal, naming colors around the room, or squeezing playdough help kids center themselves.

Adults benefit from these childlike practices, too. The more playful and non-judgmental your grounding practice, the more likely it is to stick.

Grounding in Public Spaces

You don't need a yoga mat or privacy to ground yourself. In a crowded subway, silently do the 5-4-3-2-1 method. At a noisy dinner party, focus on your breath or sip your drink slowly with attention.

Grounding is portable. It's for real life, not just quiet retreats.

The Long-Term Impact of Grounding

When practiced regularly, grounding retrains your brain and body to recognize calm as your default state. Over time, your response to stress changes. Instead of panic, you pause. Instead of spiraling, you stabilize.

You become less reactive and more responsive. Less chaotic and more clear.

Final Thoughts

Grounding isn't just a tool. It's a way of living. A lifestyle of noticing, pausing, feeling, and connecting.

We don't always have control over the storms around us. But grounding teaches us how to hold steady in the eye of the storm.

Section 4: Journaling: A Free Therapist in Your Pocket

In a world that demands constant output and digital engagement, our inner world often becomes neglected and cluttered. We consume information relentlessly but seldom pause to process it. This imbalance creates a mental bottleneck, often resulting in anxiety, confusion, and emotional fatigue. But there is a tool that doesn't require a subscription, an internet connection, or even an appointment. That tool is journaling.

Journaling is far more than a hobby. It's a powerful and profoundly simple act of self-connection. It turns vague feelings into words, chaotic thoughts into structure, and emotional turmoil into manageable reflections. It can be your sounding board, your truth-teller, your safe space. It is, quite literally, a therapist in your pocket.

The Simplicity of Self-Awareness

When you journal, you give yourself permission to pause. To listen inwardly. This act of reflection helps you move from reactivity to awareness. For many, journaling becomes the very first time in their busy day when they acknowledge their true feelings.

A study published in the *Journal of Research in Personality* revealed that people who journaled about emotional experiences reported significantly better psychological well-being, even weeks later. It is not about perfect grammar or elegant prose. It's about honesty. Journaling makes your thoughts visible so you can confront, explore, and understand them.

Think of your mind like a cluttered room. Journaling is the act of opening a window, letting fresh air in, and finally seeing the mess for what it is—so you can start to tidy it up.

Emotional Release Without Judgment

Life teaches us to suppress emotions. Anger is "ugly." Sadness is "weak." Anxiety is "overreacting." But these judgments create emotional pressure that eventually erupts—in arguments, panic attacks, burnout, or depression. Journaling offers a space where no emotion is too much.

You can be honest without hurting anyone. Angry without consequences. Vulnerable without fear. The page doesn't interrupt you. It doesn't fix or dismiss your feelings. It simply listens. And sometimes, that's all you need.

There is something almost magical about seeing your pain in ink. It softens it. It validates it. And often, it shows you that what you feared was a monster is actually a shadow needing your attention, not your avoidance.

Journaling Methods for Inner Clarity

Journaling isn't one-size-fits-all. The beauty lies in how personalized it can be. Here are a few powerful techniques:

1. Stream of Consciousness

Write without stopping, editing, or censoring. Dump everything from your mind to the page. It doesn't have to make sense. It just needs to flow. This technique is especially effective when you feel overwhelmed or mentally blocked.

Prompt: What's weighing on my mind right now?

2. Gratitude Journaling

List 3-5 things you're grateful for daily. This rewires your brain to focus on abundance rather than scarcity. It's a scientifically backed method to increase long-term happiness and reduce stress.

Prompt: What made me smile today?

3. Emotion Tracking

At the end of each day, write down how you felt and why. Over time, you'll start to notice emotional patterns. This helps you identify triggers, joys, and areas of growth.

Prompt: When did I feel most anxious or most at peace today?

4. Letters You Don't Send

Write to someone you're angry at, grieving, or missing. Say what you never got to say. These unsent letters can provide immense closure and catharsis.

Prompt: What would I say if I had no fear of judgment?

5. Vision Journaling

Dream boldly. Describe the life you want in vivid detail—emotionally, spiritually, professionally. This kind of journaling motivates and re-aligns you with your purpose.

Prompt: If fear wasn't holding me back, what would I do?

Journaling as a Daily Ritual

Consistency amplifies the benefits of journaling. It's less about writing long entries and more about creating a rhythm of checking in with yourself. Just five to ten minutes a day can shift your mindset, reduce stress, and build emotional intelligence.

Set the stage for your journaling practice:

- Find a quiet corner.
- Light a candle or play soft music.
- Use a pen you enjoy writing with.
- Choose a notebook that feels inviting.

Let it become your sanctuary—not a task, but a sacred habit.

If digital journaling works better for you (say, through apps like Day One or Notion), go for it. The medium doesn't matter. The intention does.

Journaling and Mental Health

Mental health professionals often use journaling as part of cognitive-behavioral therapy (CBT). It helps clients recognize negative thought loops, challenge unhelpful beliefs, and track emotional shifts. Even without a therapist, journaling acts as a gentle, self-led practice of mental hygiene.

In fact, during high-stress events—a breakup, a career transition, a pandemic—journaling becomes a lifeline. It helps regulate your nervous system, process trauma, and provide a record of how you made it through. When you look back, you'll often find evidence of growth you never noticed in the moment.

When You Don't Know What to Write

Sometimes, the hardest part is starting. Here are a few gentle prompts to break the blank page:

- What did I learn about myself today?
- What's one thing I'm avoiding, and why?
- What's something I need to hear right now?
- If I met my younger self, what would I say to them?
- What's something I'm proud of today?

There's no wrong way to journal. There's only your way. And every entry, no matter how short or messy, is a thread in the tapestry of your healing.

The Gentle Revolution Within

You don't need to go on a week-long retreat or delete all your social media accounts to find peace. Journaling is a micro-act with macro impact. It brings you back to yourself. It reminds you that you have wisdom, clarity, and strength inside you—you just need a moment to listen.

By turning your gaze inward regularly, you create space. Space for healing. Space for intention. Space for truth.

And in a world that constantly tells you to broadcast everything, journaling invites you to become beautifully, unapologetically private. A sacred rebel of the soul.

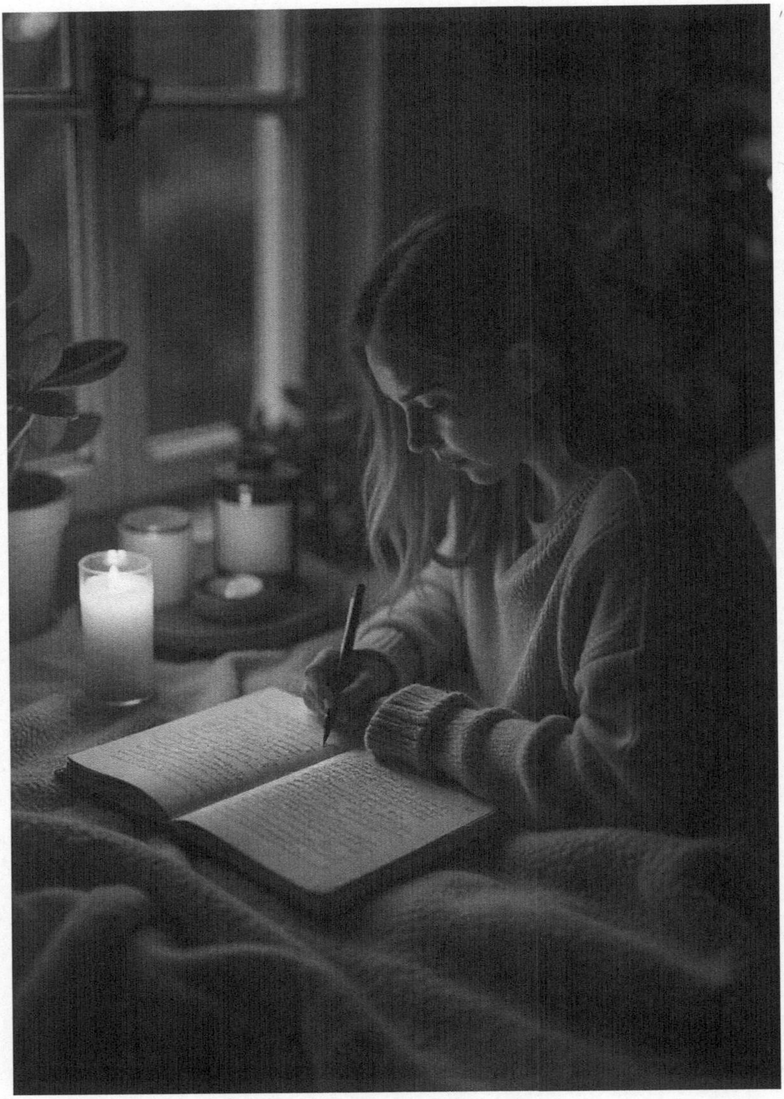

Section 5: When to Meditate (and When It's Okay Not To)

The world has been swept up by the meditation movement. From mobile apps and guided YouTube sessions to workplace wellness programs, meditation is now promoted almost everywhere as the solution for stress, anxiety, and the modern mind. While meditation is indeed a powerful tool, what is often overlooked in all the excitement is the pressure it can bring — especially when you feel like you're not doing it "right," or that you have to do it at all.

This chapter explores not only when to meditate, but more importantly, when it's okay not to. Mental quiet is not reserved for those who sit cross-legged in perfect silence. Peace is personal, and your path to it doesn't have to match anyone else's.

The Idealized Image of Meditation

Let's start by addressing the idealized version of meditation that we see everywhere: someone sitting cross-legged on a beach at sunrise, eyes closed, back straight, completely serene. While this image is inspiring, it also creates unrealistic expectations. Meditation, at its core, is about mindfulness, awareness, and stillness. You don't need the ocean, incense, or perfect posture to access these.

For some people, sitting still and breathing in silence is incredibly soothing. For others, it can feel suffocating, especially when their minds are in overdrive. And that's okay. We are all wired differently.

When Meditation Truly Helps

Meditation is a fantastic reset button for your nervous system, especially in the following moments:

- **When you're feeling overwhelmed**: Even a 2-minute breathing pause can shift your state.
- **Before or after a big transition**: Like starting your day, preparing for a difficult conversation, or winding down before sleep.
- **When you're disconnected from your body**: Meditation brings you back to the here and now.
- **As a daily ritual**: For many, just 5-10 minutes each morning helps them feel grounded and present.

You can start by focusing on your breath, or just noticing sounds, smells, and sensations around you. The aim is not to "empty" the mind but to **become aware** of it without judgment.

Remember, consistency matters more than duration. Even one minute of presence can be transformative if practiced regularly.

When Meditation Might Not Be the Answer

This might sound controversial in wellness spaces, but it needs to be said: meditation isn't always the right tool for everyone, especially not in every moment.

- **When your body is in a trauma response**: Trying to sit still while in a fight-or-flight state can make things worse. In these moments, grounding through movement, talking, or even crying may be more effective.

- **When you feel pressured to do it perfectly**: Meditation should never become another to-do or performance metric.
- **When it becomes escapism**: Sometimes we use meditation to avoid hard emotions or conversations. In those moments, honest reflection or support from a friend or therapist may help more.
- **When you're already emotionally regulated**: You don't always need to meditate. Some days, simply enjoying a quiet walk or a deep laugh can be your moment of presence.

If sitting in silence increases your anxiety, it doesn't mean you're broken. It means your system is asking for another kind of support first. Meditation is a tool, not a moral standard.

Alternatives That Work Just as Well

So, what can you do when meditation doesn't feel right? Here are practical, body-friendly alternatives that also create mental quiet:

1. **Walking Meditation**: Go for a slow, intentional walk. Focus on the movement of your feet, the sounds around you, the wind on your skin.
2. **Creative Expression**: Drawing, painting, baking, knitting, or even gardening can be deeply meditative.
3. **Body Scanning**: Lie down and gently bring awareness to different parts of your body, noticing tension and letting go.

4. **Prayer or Devotional Time**: For many, prayer offers both reflection and emotional release.
5. **Listening to Music Mindfully**: Put on an instrumental piece and focus on each sound, each pause.

What matters most is that the practice makes you feel *more* present and peaceful, not more anxious or ashamed.

Real-Life Stories

Lena, 34, Teacher: "I tried meditating every morning because everyone said it would help my anxiety. But I found myself dreading it. Then I switched to journaling while sipping tea on my balcony. That's my peace now."

Raj, 42, Engineer: "Meditation helped me for a while, but during a period of burnout, it felt impossible. What helped was walking in the park and listening to nature. Later, I returned to meditation naturally."

These stories show that mindfulness isn't a one-size-fits-all approach. It's a fluid, flexible relationship with your inner world.

Tips for Making Meditation Work for You

If you do want to build a meditation practice that works, try these:

- **Start with small, achievable goals**: Just 2-3 minutes a day is enough.

- **Use guided meditations**: Apps like Insight Timer, Calm, or Headspace can help.
- **Change positions**: Try lying down, standing, or even meditating while doing gentle chores.
- **Release the need for silence**: Some people prefer meditating with background music, nature sounds, or affirmations.
- **Be kind to your mind**: Thoughts will come. The goal is not to stop them but to watch them pass like clouds.

Releasing the Guilt

Above all, let go of guilt. There is no spiritual scoreboard. You don't need to meditate to be a good person or to prove you are healing.

If meditation feels right today, do it. If not, that's also okay. Inner peace is built through honesty, not obligation.

Your worth is not measured by your ability to sit still in silence.

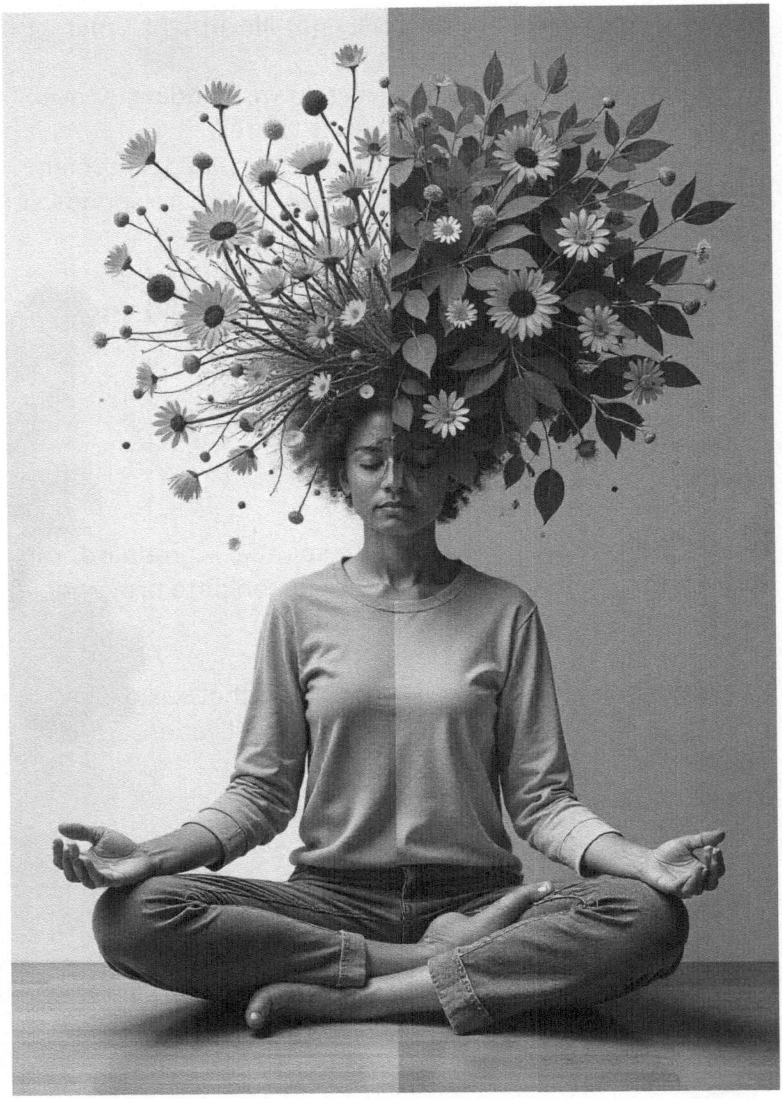

Section 6: Replacing Overthinking with Curiosity

We often associate overthinking with intelligence. We assume that a mind running in circles is a mind that's engaged, productive, and preparing for what's ahead. But the truth is far from it. Overthinking rarely leads to clarity. Instead, it creates fog, confusion, and emotional exhaustion. It disconnects us from the present and traps us in a loop of imagined problems and hypothetical scenarios.

What if we told you that the antidote to overthinking isn't logic, but curiosity?

Let's begin by reframing what's happening when we overthink. At its core, overthinking is often a protective mechanism. Our minds go into overdrive trying to predict, prevent, or perfect. We rehash conversations. We imagine what could go wrong. We analyze decisions until all our mental energy is gone—and still, no answer feels good enough.

Overthinking stems from fear: fear of failure, fear of regret, fear of not being enough. It masquerades as control but creates the exact opposite—mental chaos.

From Mental Loops to Mental Expansion

Curiosity, on the other hand, invites us into the present with wonder. It doesn't demand perfect answers. It just asks, "What can I notice? What else might be true? What might happen if I try something different?" Curiosity invites growth, learning, and freedom. It doesn't shut down possibilities. It opens them.

Imagine you're facing a challenging decision—maybe about changing careers, starting a business, or moving to a new city. An overthinking mindset might say:

- "What if it doesn't work out?"
- "What if I'm making a huge mistake?"
- "What will others think?"

A curious mindset reframes:

- "What could I learn from trying this?"
- "What excites me about this possibility?"
- "What small step can I take to explore this further?"

Curiosity grounds us in inquiry instead of fear. It allows us to acknowledge risk without letting risk control us. It shifts us from paralysis to playful exploration.

Everyday Curiosity Tools

So how do we practice this mental shift? Here are some simple daily tools you can incorporate:

1. Ask Better Questions

Start noticing the kinds of questions you ask yourself. Are they fear-based or growth-based?

- Fear-based: "Why am I like this?" "What if it all goes wrong?"
- Growth-based: "What am I learning from this?" "What would I try if I weren't afraid?"

Switching your internal questions can change the emotional tone of your inner dialogue.

2. Get Playful with Mistakes

Overthinkers often fear failure. They catastrophize mistakes. But curiosity sees mistakes as feedback. Like a scientist in a lab, it says: “Interesting result! What can I learn from this?”

Try reframing your errors:

- "That didn’t go as planned—what might I try next time?"
- "That was tough—what helped me get through it?"

3. Use the "Maybe" Mind

In mindfulness practices, there's a concept called "Beginner’s Mind." It means seeing things with fresh eyes, like a child seeing snow for the first time. Rather than assuming you know what will happen, try thinking:

- "Maybe this will be different."
- "Maybe this is an opportunity."
- "Maybe I don’t have to have it all figured out."

"Maybe" helps loosen the grip of certainty and perfectionism.

4. Journaling with Curiosity

Journaling can become a powerful tool to practice curiosity. Try using prompts like:

- "What am I curious about today?"
- "What surprised me recently?"
- "What assumptions am I making right now?"

These questions invite exploration rather than analysis. Over time, they can rewire your thought patterns.

5. Practice Presence in Micro-Moments

Curiosity thrives in presence. When you're overthinking, you're usually mentally elsewhere—in the past or in the future. Practice grounding yourself in the now.

Try:

- Noticing five new things around you
- Taking a slow breath and asking, "What do I feel right now?"
- Tuning in to your senses without judgment (sight, sound, smell, taste, touch)

These grounding moments calm your nervous system and open space for curiosity to rise.

Overthinking vs. Curiosity: A Side-by-Side

Overthinking	**Curiosity**
Driven by fear and control	Driven by wonder and openness
Seeks certainty and perfection	Embraces learning and experimentation
Paralysis through analysis	Movement through exploration
Often rigid and repetitive	Flexible and imaginative
Drains emotional energy	Inspires emotional resilience

Replacing "Why Me?" with "What's Next?"

One subtle but powerful shift is moving from “Why?” to “What now?”

Overthinking often asks: “Why did this happen to me?” “Why can’t I get this right?”

Curiosity asks: “What’s my next best step?” “What else can I try?”

The first keeps you spinning. The second moves you forward.

A Word on Self-Compassion

Curiosity isn’t a performance. It’s a practice. You’re allowed to be scared, confused, and tired. You don’t need to have all the answers. You just need a willingness to keep asking kind, open-hearted questions.

When you catch yourself in an overthinking loop, take a breath and whisper: “I wonder what else is possible?” That one question can break the cycle.

Chapter 5 Summary: Finding Mental Quiet in a Loud World

In a world that rarely stops talking, Chapter 5 helped us discover how to quiet our minds. We began by unpacking **what mental noise really is**—the swirl of thoughts, expectations, and distractions that keeps us anxious and disconnected. We then learned the power of **present moment awareness**, how it anchors us in peace, and the value of **simple grounding practices** that anyone can integrate into their day.

We explored the reflective power of **journaling**, our free and portable therapist, and we gave meditation a human touch—reminding ourselves that it's not a requirement but an invitation. Finally, in this section, we explored how **replacing overthinking with curiosity** transforms our mental landscape from one of fear to one of exploration, growth, and gentleness.

When we quiet the noise and come home to ourselves, peace isn't somewhere far away—it's right here, waiting in the pause.

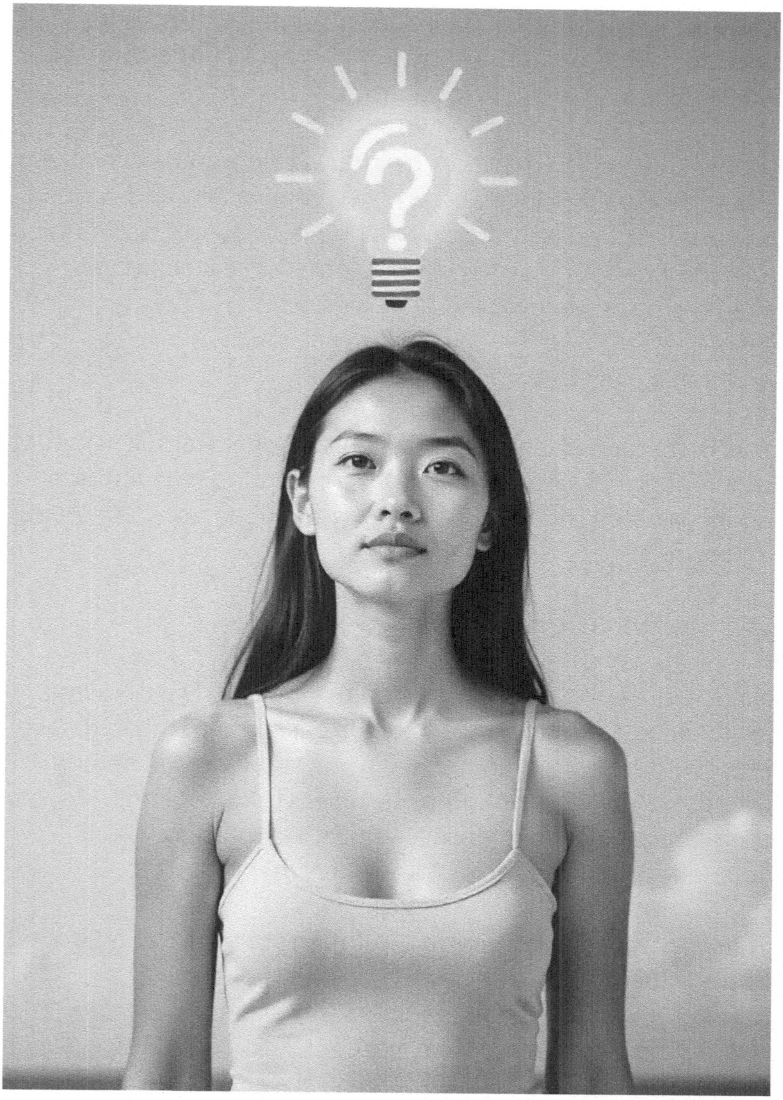

Chapter 6: Healing Relationships, Setting Boundaries
Section 1: People Can Be Draining — and That's Okay to Admit

We live in a world where connection is celebrated—where we are encouraged to love fiercely, give generously, and support one another tirelessly. Yet in this noble pursuit of community and compassion, we often forget something vital: people, even the ones we love, can be draining.

And that's okay to admit.

This isn't about villainizing others or building walls. It's about reclaiming your emotional energy, respecting your limits, and understanding that being a kind person does not mean being a doormat.

The Hidden Cost of Constant Availability

Have you ever left a conversation feeling utterly exhausted, as if your soul had been rung dry like a sponge? It could have been with a family member, a coworker, or even a lifelong friend. Maybe their problems became your problems. Maybe their energy was so intense, so negative, that you found yourself feeling low without knowing why.

These moments are common, yet many of us are conditioned to push them aside. "Be strong," we're told. "Be there for others." But emotional exhaustion is real, and pretending it isn't only buries the problem deeper.

People-pleasing, over-giving, and being the go-to listener for everyone else's crisis may sound like good character. And while empathy is a beautiful trait, unmanaged empathy can lead to burnout, resentment, and even anxiety. Sometimes, the people who drain us the most are those we feel most obligated to help.

Emotional Vampires Exist (Even If They're Unaware)

The term "emotional vampire" might sound harsh, but it accurately describes someone who unconsciously or deliberately sucks the energy out of you. This could be a chronic complainer, a drama magnet, a manipulator, or someone who always "needs you" but is never there when you need them.

These aren't always toxic people in the classic sense. Often, they're hurting. They may not mean to drain others, but their unprocessed emotions, neediness, or lack of boundaries force you into roles you never signed up for: therapist, rescuer, peacekeeper.

You are not obligated to carry what they refuse to process.

Guilt vs. Compassion

A huge reason many of us allow this emotional draining to continue is guilt.

Guilt whispers, "If you were a good person, you wouldn't walk away."

But compassion whispers something else entirely: "You can love people and still choose to protect your peace."

Here's a truth you need to hear—**you are not responsible for managing anyone else's emotions but your own**. There is a stark difference between being supportive and being emotionally entangled. One brings growth; the other brings depletion.

How to Identify Draining Relationships

Not all draining people are obvious. Sometimes, it's subtle. Here are signs someone may be draining your energy:

- You feel anxious or heavy before or after talking to them.
- You feel obligated to respond immediately to their texts or calls.
- They never ask how *you* are, or they quickly redirect the conversation back to themselves.
- You're constantly solving their problems.
- You feel guilty when you don't engage.

Take a moment to reflect: who leaves you feeling energized and who leaves you feeling empty? Our bodies are wise. They keep score.

You Are Allowed to Protect Your Energy

There is profound courage in admitting that some relationships are not healthy for your well-being. This doesn't mean cutting everyone off or becoming emotionally distant. It means learning the art of boundaries.

Protecting your energy isn't selfish. It's self-respect.

Ask yourself:

- Can I be kind and still say "I can't help right now"?
- Can I support someone without absorbing their pain?
- Can I choose distance without shame?

The answer to all of these is a powerful **yes**.

Boundaries Are Not Walls; They Are Bridges

Boundaries are not about pushing people away. They are about bringing healthier versions of ourselves into every relationship.

Consider this:

- Saying "no" to a coffee date with a draining friend doesn't make you a bad person.
- Not picking up the phone at 11 PM doesn't make you unloving.
- Choosing silence over small talk doesn't make you cold.

These choices create space for restoration. And in that space, we begin to find peace.

Navigating Guilt, Resistance, and Pushback

When you start setting boundaries, you may get pushback. Especially from people who have benefited from your lack of boundaries.

That's not a sign you're doing it wrong—it's a sign you're doing it right.

If someone truly loves you, they will adjust. They may not understand at first, but real love is not built on access; it is built on respect.

Start small:

- Delay your response to non-urgent texts.
- Take breaks from conversations that feel one-sided.
- Practice saying, "I'm not available for that right now."

With time, you'll find that these small steps create profound shifts.

The Beauty of Restored Energy

When you stop leaking your emotional energy into draining interactions, something amazing happens: you come back to yourself.

Your mind clears. Your sleep deepens. Your creativity flows. Your joy returns.

This is what protecting your peace looks like in action. You are no longer spending energy defending your needs. You are simply living them.

Imagine waking up without dread, walking through your day with lightness, and having the capacity to offer others your *best*, not just your leftovers. That's what happens when we stop pouring from an empty cup.

Final Thought: It's Okay to Choose You

Sometimes healing begins not with more giving, but with less. Not with more connection, but with more solitude. Choosing yourself may be uncomfortable at first—especially if you're used to over-giving. But in choosing yourself, you teach others to do the same.

Give yourself permission to say:

- "I love you, but I need space."
- "I care, but I can't carry this."
- "I matter too."

Because you do.

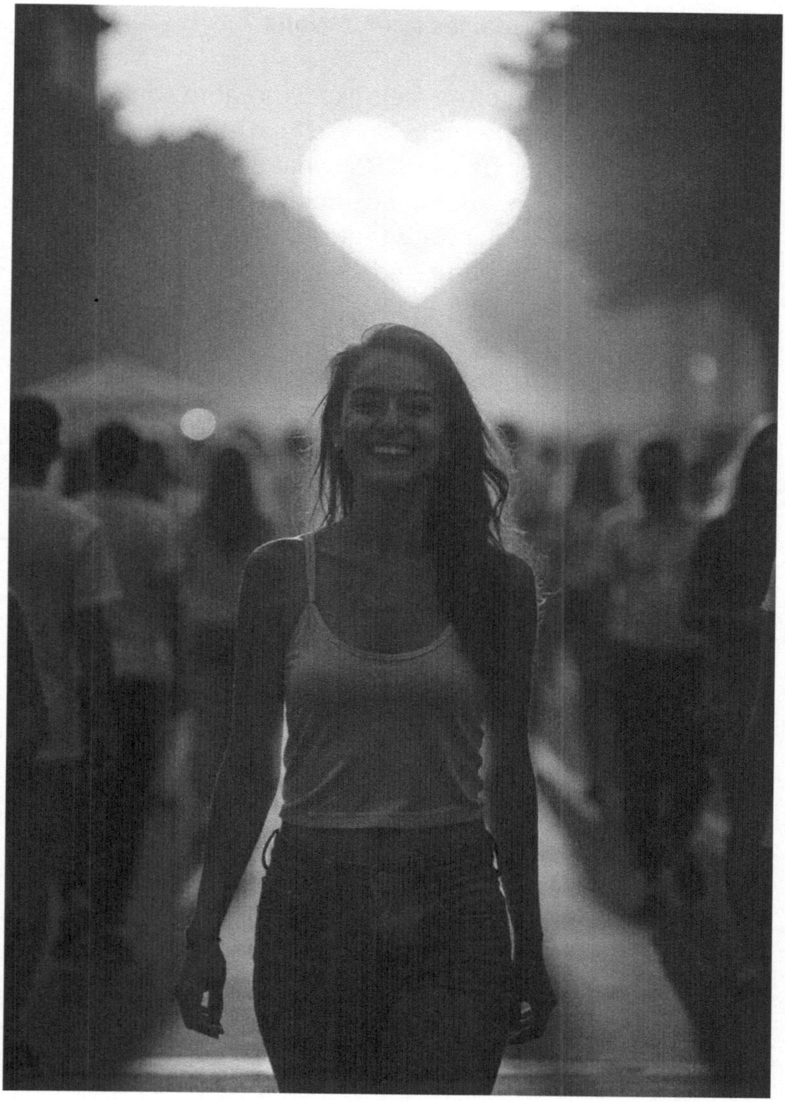

Section 2: Why Boundaries Aren't Walls

Boundaries. The word often feels like a threat to connection. In cultures that value harmony and self-sacrifice, setting a boundary can feel like betrayal. But what if boundaries aren't the end of connection, but the beginning of healthier ones? What if boundaries aren't walls that shut people out, but bridges that help both parties cross over into respect, compassion, and clarity?

Let's reframe the conversation. Let's stop imagining boundaries as high, cold walls built out of anger or fear. Instead, picture a garden. A garden with a little wooden fence around it. Not to keep people away, but to protect what is precious inside. The boundary says, "You are welcome here, but please use the gate, and wipe your feet."

The Truth About Boundaries

Boundaries are not about rejecting people. They are about rejecting behavior that wounds, drains, or disrespects. You can deeply love someone and still need space from them. You can be committed to your family and still say "no." Boundaries allow you to remain in relationship *without* losing yourself.

The key difference between a boundary and a wall is intention. A boundary invites conversation. A wall avoids it. A boundary honors your needs. A wall hides them. Boundaries say, "I love you and I love me, so let's figure out how we can both thrive."

Here are a few truths to guide us:

- **Boundaries are proactive, not reactive.**
- **Boundaries are about clarity, not control.**

- **Boundaries are expressions of self-respect.**

Boundaries vs. Walls: Understanding the Difference

Feature	Boundaries	Walls
Motivation	Protection and clarity	Fear or avoidance
Communication	Open, respectful dialogue	Silence or passive-aggression
Purpose	Preserve connection while honoring needs	Sever connection to avoid vulnerability
Impact	Builds healthier relationships	Causes isolation and misunderstanding

Consider the difference in a real-world example:

Boundary: "I would love to talk with you, but I can't take calls after 9 PM anymore. That's my wind-down time. Can we chat tomorrow instead?"

Wall: Not answering the phone, turning off notifications, and growing resentful without explanation.

One builds trust and clarity. The other builds distance and confusion.

Why We Fear Setting Boundaries

Let's be honest: boundaries feel scary because they often trigger guilt, especially if you were raised to equate love with sacrifice. Many of us grew up with the message that good people say "yes," that being available equals being kind.

But what if being kind to others meant being cruel to yourself? That's not love—that's emotional erasure.

When you first start setting boundaries, people might resist. That's not necessarily because you're doing something wrong—it might be because they're used to you having none.

Remember:

- People who benefit from your lack of boundaries are often the ones who push back when you set them.
- Discomfort is not a sign that your boundary is wrong—it's often a sign that it's needed.

Think of it as renovating a house: it gets messy before it gets better.

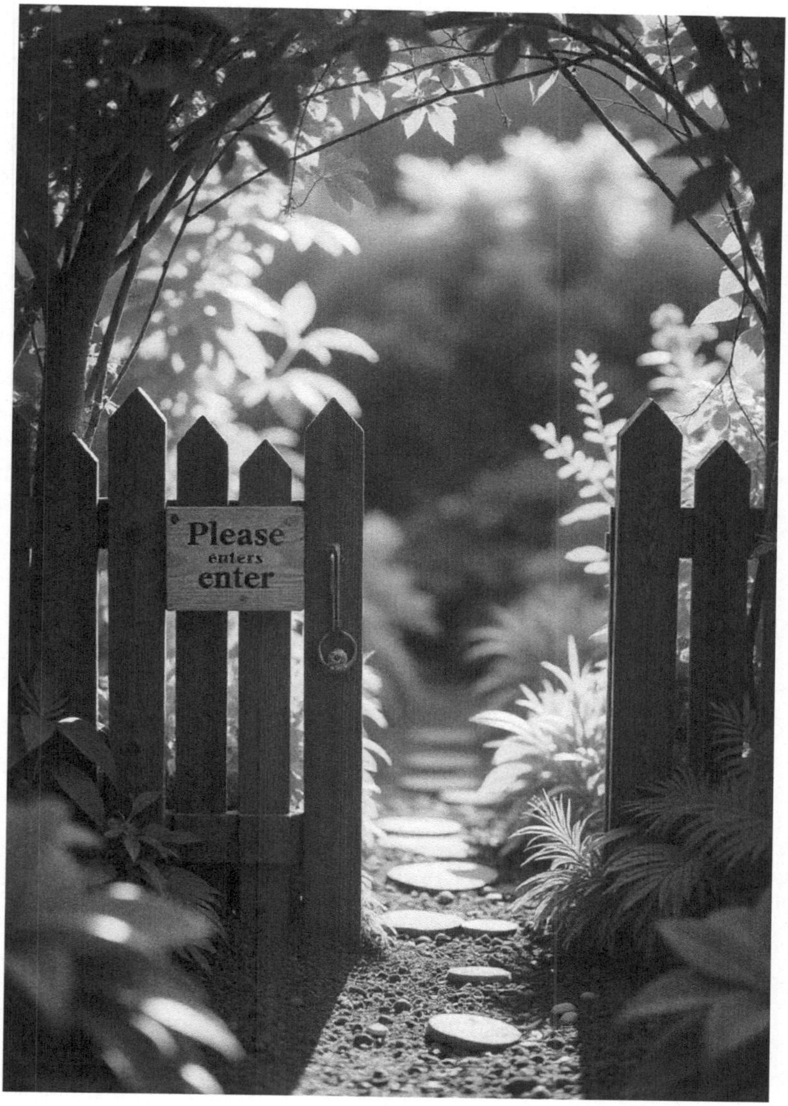
Please
enters
enter

Rewriting the Script: Healthy Boundary Statements

Boundaries don't need to be harsh to be firm. They can be kind and clear.

Here are a few examples:

- "I'm not available to talk right now, but I care about you and will check in later."
- "I'm not comfortable with that topic. Let's talk about something else."
- "I want to help, but I can't commit to that right now."
- "I need some alone time to recharge. I'll reach out when I'm ready."

These statements express love, presence, and clarity. They don't accuse or attack. They simply inform others about your emotional and energetic limits.

Remember, a person who respects your boundary is a person who respects *you*.

When Boundaries Are Mistaken for Rejection

It's common for people to misinterpret boundaries, especially if they're not used to them. If someone says, "You've changed," it might mean you've stopped abandoning yourself.

This is where courage steps in. You must decide what matters more: keeping the peace externally or creating peace internally. One is temporary. The other is lasting.

If someone walks away because you asked for respect, they were never truly invested in your well-being. Real connection survives honesty. It may not always feel good in the moment, but it *builds* over time.

The Ripple Effect of Boundaries

Setting boundaries is like tossing a stone into a pond. The ripples affect everything around you:

- Your kids learn what self-respect looks like.
- Your friendships become more balanced.
- Your body feels less drained and more energized.
- You start attracting people who don't just want access to you, but want *relationship* with you.

And the biggest ripple? You begin to trust yourself.

When you know your limits, you no longer live in fear of being used, walked over, or misunderstood. You carry a quiet strength. That strength brings peace.

When Boundaries Are Spiritual

Let's not forget: even Jesus had boundaries. He withdrew from the crowds. He said "no." He rested. He didn't say "yes" to every request or demand.

Setting a boundary is not selfish—it's sacred. It is an act of stewardship over your energy, your mental health, and your calling.

Whether you come from a faith background or not, the principle remains: we are human. Finite. We are not machines, endlessly available. Boundaries help us live as we were designed to—with intention, rhythm, and care.

The Gentle Art of Holding the Line

Not every boundary needs a speech. Sometimes, it's in your tone. Your schedule. Your decisions. Boundaries are less about pushing others away and more about pulling yourself inward—to truth, to clarity, to self-respect.

Here's a final tip:

Boundaries are not just spoken. They're lived.

When your calendar reflects your values, when your conversations reflect your capacity, when your rest is protected—you don't need to constantly defend your boundaries. They become the quiet language of how you love yourself.

And others learn to listen.

Section 3: How to Set Limits Without Feeling Guilty

If you've ever found yourself agreeing to something you didn't want to do, staying in a conversation that made you feel drained, or continuing a relationship that caused more pain than joy, you're not alone. Many of us have been conditioned to associate setting boundaries with being selfish, rude, or uncaring. But boundaries are not barriers. They are bridges to healthier versions of ourselves and our relationships. This section is about learning how to set those limits clearly, confidently, and without guilt.

Why We Struggle With Guilt When Setting Limits

Guilt creeps in because most of us grew up being taught that good people say yes, help out, and put others first. While kindness and compassion are virtues, they should not come at the cost of our mental, emotional, or physical health.

When we start asserting boundaries, it can feel like we're violating those internal rules. We worry about hurting others, being misunderstood, or coming across as cold. Often, this guilt is less about the boundary itself and more about a fear of disconnection.

Here's the truth: you can love people deeply and still say no. You can care and still walk away. Protecting your peace is not selfish—it's essential.

Reframing the Role of Boundaries

Before diving into the how-to, it helps to reframe what boundaries are:

- **Boundaries are a form of communication, not confrontation.**
- **Boundaries are an act of self-respect, not rejection of others.**
- **Boundaries are tools for clarity, not weapons of control.**

When you see them through this lens, setting limits becomes less about shutting people out and more about letting them in the right way—with honesty, respect, and clear expectations.

Practical Ways to Set Limits Without Feeling Guilty

1. **Know Your Non-Negotiables**

   Begin by identifying what truly matters to you. Is it your sleep schedule? Your weekend rest? The time you spend with your family? Your emotional safety?

   Create a short list of non-negotiables—things you will not compromise on. Knowing these will help you feel justified when you have to say no or make a choice that prioritizes your well-being.

2. **Use Gentle But Firm Language**

   You can be kind and assertive at the same time. Here are some example phrases:

   - "I appreciate the invite, but I need time to recharge."
   - "I understand you're disappointed, but I can't commit to that right now."
   - "This doesn't work for me, but I hope you find the support you need."

   Language matters. You don't owe anyone long explanations. A simple, clear statement can be powerful.

3. **Practice With Low-Stakes Situations**

   Start small. Practice setting boundaries in less emotionally loaded situations, like declining a social gathering, asking for extra time on a task, or requesting a quieter workspace.

These smaller actions build your confidence and prepare you for bigger conversations.

4. **Expect Resistance and Don't Personalize It**

   When you set a new limit, others may push back—especially if they've benefited from your lack of boundaries in the past. This doesn't mean you're doing something wrong. It often means you're doing something necessary.

   People may respond with confusion, frustration, or guilt-tripping. Recognize this as a reflection of their discomfort with change, not your wrongdoing.

5. **Build a Support System**

   Surround yourself with people who respect your boundaries and encourage your growth. Share your journey with trusted friends or a therapist who can affirm your right to take up space in your life.

   When you're unsure, having someone to validate your decision can ease the guilt.

6. **Reconnect With Your Body During Boundary-Setting**

   Pay attention to physical cues. Do you feel tension in your shoulders, tightness in your jaw, or a pit in your stomach when you're about to say yes but want to say no?

   These signals are valuable. Take a breath, pause, and make a choice from a place of calm.

7. **Celebrate Small Wins**

   Every time you set a boundary, acknowledge it. Write it down in a journal. Tell a friend. Sit with the feeling of empowerment it brings.

   Over time, these victories compound, and guilt fades into a quiet confidence.

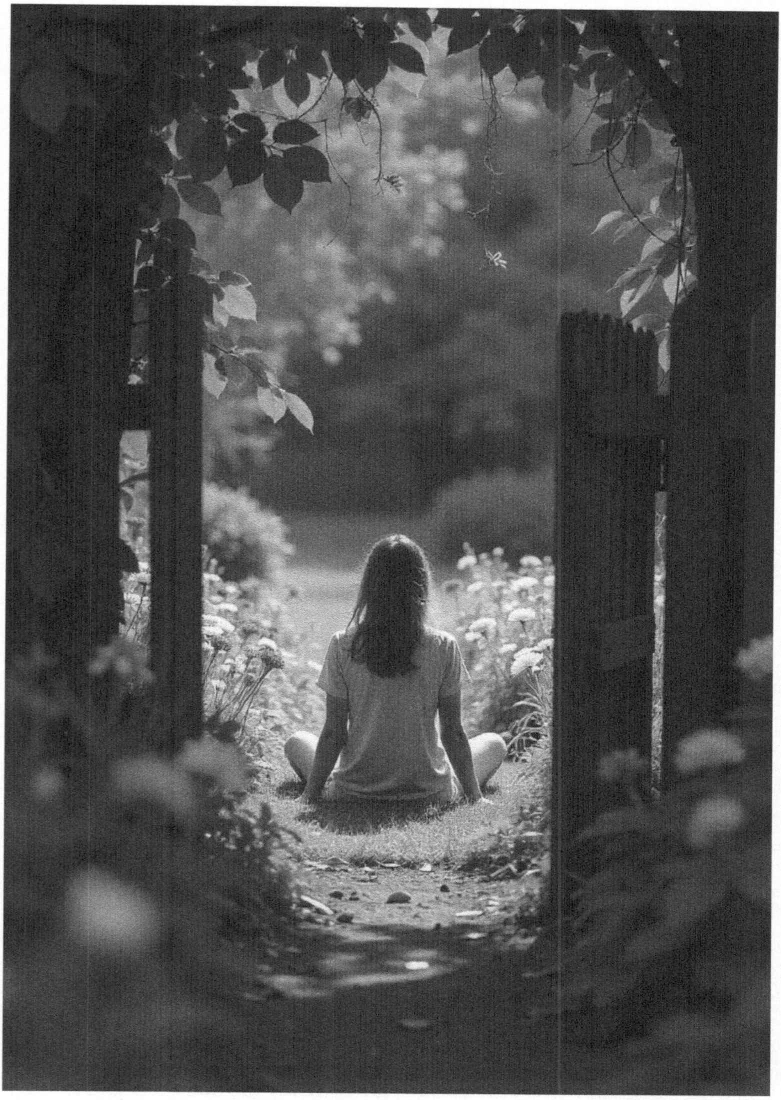

When Guilt Persists: A Gentle Reminder

If guilt continues to show up even after practice, pause and ask yourself:

- Am I betraying myself to please someone else?
- Will saying yes cause me stress, resentment, or burnout?
- What would I tell a loved one in the same situation?

Most of the time, we're much kinder to others than to ourselves. You deserve the same compassion and protection you offer so freely to everyone else.

The Emotional Cost of Boundary Avoidance

When you don't set boundaries, the cost is often silent but steep:

- Chronic fatigue
- Emotional resentment
- Strained relationships
- Identity loss
- Poor mental health

Setting limits is not about keeping others out; it's about keeping yourself intact.

Final Thoughts: Guilt Is a Sign of Growth

If you feel guilty after setting a boundary, see it as a growing pain. It means you're unlearning unhealthy patterns and stepping into a new way of being. Be patient with yourself.

Think of guilt as an old coat you wore to keep others warm. Now, you're realizing it no longer fits. It's time to put on something that warms you, too.

Section 4: Having the Hard Conversations With Calm

In every human relationship, there comes a time when words must carry weight. Conversations about unmet needs, disappointments, shifting expectations, or deeply personal boundaries aren't just necessary—they are unavoidable. And yet, most of us delay or avoid these hard conversations because we fear conflict, rejection, or the emotional intensity they may stir.

But here is a truth often hidden beneath our hesitation: avoiding hard conversations doesn't preserve peace; it only prolongs discomfort. When we learn to have these talks with calm, clarity, and compassion, we create space for truth, healing, and authentic connection.

Why Hard Conversations Are So Hard

It's not just what we say, but what we fear might happen as a result. For many of us, challenging conversations trigger a flight-or-fight response. We fear that we might hurt someone, ruin a relationship, or be dismissed altogether. Cultural conditioning plays a role here, especially in environments where maintaining harmony is valued more than voicing individual needs.

We also carry emotional baggage into these moments—past experiences where we weren't heard, or where vulnerability was met with judgment or dismissal. That emotional residue makes every new difficult conversation feel like a potential landmine.

The Calm Before the Talk: Preparing Internally

To approach hard conversations with calm, the internal preparation is just as important as the words you plan to say. Consider this an emotional reset:

1. **Get Clear on the Purpose**: Are you setting a boundary, expressing a need, or seeking clarity? Knowing your purpose helps prevent spiraling into blame or vague frustration.
2. **Check Your Emotional Temperature**: If you're angry, hurt, or overwhelmed, wait. Process those emotions first. Go for a walk. Journal. Pray. Breathe. A regulated nervous system is your greatest ally in a high-stakes conversation.
3. **Release the Outcome**: You can't control how the other person will respond. But you can control your tone, your clarity, and your composure. Speaking truth is your responsibility—accepting it is theirs.
4. **Practice**: Say it out loud in front of a mirror or record yourself. This isn't about memorization, but about finding the most grounded, calm version of your message.

Creating the Right Environment

Setting matters. Aim for privacy, a calm setting, and a time when neither of you is hungry, rushed, or emotionally depleted. Avoid texting or emailing tough topics if the subject deserves face-to-face communication.

You can begin with an intention: *"I want to share something that matters to me, and I hope we can talk about it calmly."* Let your tone mirror your purpose. A soft voice can carry even the hardest truths.

The Anatomy of a Hard Conversation

A helpful structure can anchor you:

1. **Observation Without Blame**: Start with what happened, not what you assume they meant. "I noticed that you've canceled the last few times we planned to meet."
2. **Share How It Affected You**: This is not about guilt-tripping but revealing your internal world. "It left me feeling unimportant and unsure about our friendship."
3. **State Your Need or Request**: Get clear on what you hope changes. "It would mean a lot to me if we could plan something and stick to it—and if that's not possible, I'd love to understand why."

This structure turns confrontation into communication. It opens a door rather than draws a line.

Dealing With Defensiveness or Pushback

Not everyone is ready for truth. Some people deflect, deny, or shut down. That's not your fault. Stay calm. Repeat your message gently if needed. You can say:

- "I'm not trying to blame you. I just want to share how I feel so we can understand each other better."
- "If this feels like a lot, I'm okay taking a break and coming back to it."

Your calm is contagious. When you stay regulated, you offer a blueprint for others to do the same.

What If the Conversation Changes the Relationship?

That's possible. It might lead to a deepening of understanding or a redefining of closeness. Some relationships evolve. Others fade. But each hard conversation refines your alignment with peace and authenticity.

Hard conversations may cause temporary discomfort, but they protect your long-term well-being.

Biblical Wisdom for Hard Conversations

Scripture doesn't avoid conflict; it teaches us how to navigate it with grace. Proverbs 15:1 says, *"A gentle answer turns away wrath, but a harsh word stirs up anger."* Christ modeled truth-telling wrapped in love, confronting wrongs without condemnation, and inviting reflection rather than defensiveness.

Let your conversations be rooted in love, not ego. Approach with humility, and remember, speaking the truth in love is a spiritual discipline.

The Gift of Emotional Honesty

Being honest about your feelings is not selfish—it's sacred. When done calmly, emotional honesty builds bridges instead of walls. It gives others a chance to rise to the occasion and meet you where you are.

And even if they don't, you walk away knowing you stood in your truth without losing your peace.

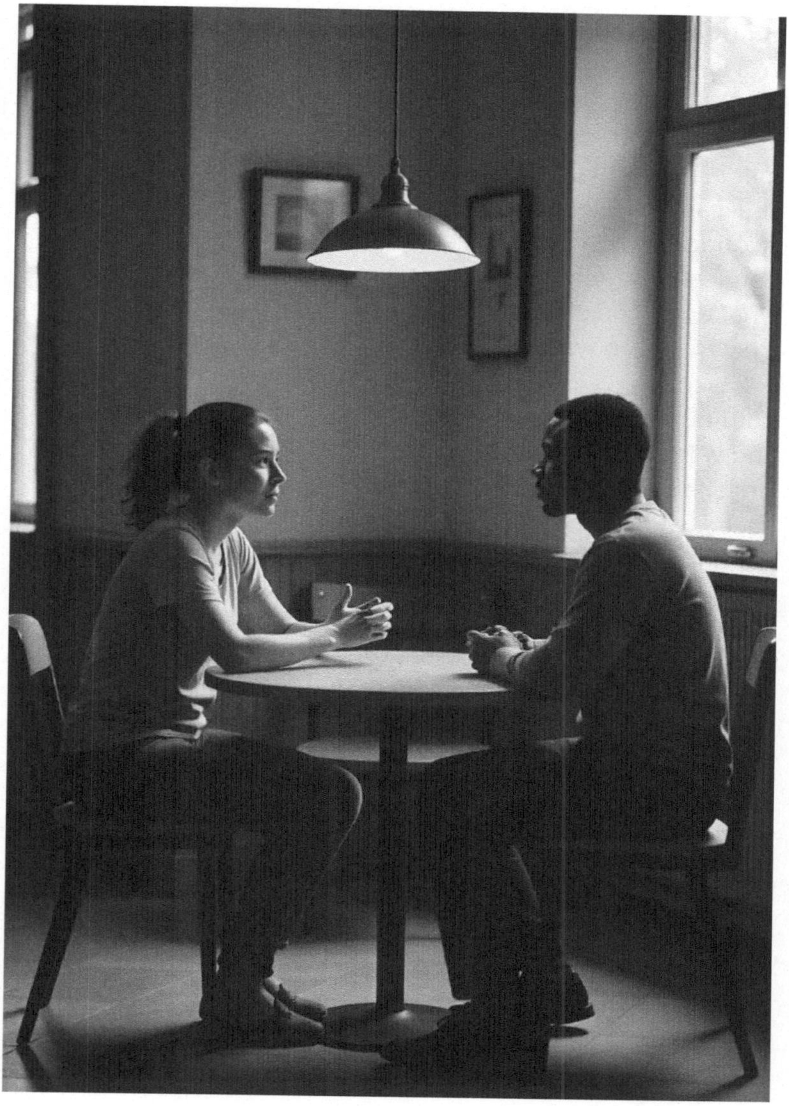

Section 5: Finding "Your People" in a Loud, Crowded World

In a world that celebrates extroversion, popularity, and social media highlights, finding people who truly resonate with your soul can feel like looking for a needle in a haystack. The world is louder than ever. Between buzzing phones, constant notifications, and the ever-present pressure to keep up with what everyone else is doing, it can be hard to discern who is truly meant to walk with you through life.

But finding your people—the ones who see you, hear you, and value you just as you are—isn't about having the biggest circle. It's about having an honest one. And in today's fast-paced, connection-saturated culture, building deep, authentic relationships can feel rare, even impossible.

Why It Feels So Hard

Many of us grow up learning how to blend in. We learn to say what others want to hear, to smooth over our edges, to be agreeable. Over time, we can lose touch with who we really are, let alone know who truly sees us. We might spend years with people who know our social masks but have no idea what keeps us awake at night or lights our soul on fire.

Add to this the curated perfection of social media, where friendship is measured by "likes" and presence is filtered for aesthetics, and it's easy to feel like everyone else has their tribe—except you.

But the truth is, you don't need hundreds of people. You need the right few. And they may not come easily or quickly, but they are out there. Finding them starts with one essential step: being radically, unapologetically yourself.

Becoming Who You Are So You Can Be Found

You attract what you reflect. If you're hiding parts of yourself to gain approval or fit in, you'll likely connect with people who are doing the same. Those connections often feel shallow, temporary, and unfulfilling.

But when you show up as your real self—quirks, boundaries, values, and all—you send a signal. You let others know who you are and what you stand for. And in doing so, you make it easier for your people to find you.

This may mean saying "no" to things that once made you feel included but now feel exhausting. It may mean walking away from groups where you feel you must earn love instead of simply being loved. This isn't selfishness. It's self-respect.

The Quiet Power of Small Circles

There is something deeply grounding about knowing you don't need to please a crowd. Intimacy doesn't grow in crowds. It grows in consistency, presence, and vulnerability.

Your people are the ones who:

- Listen without fixing.
- Celebrate your wins without competition.
- Respect your "no" without guilt-tripping you.
- Support your healing, not your image.

You don't have to explain yourself constantly to them. There's an ease in their presence. And yes, you might only have two or three of them. But when the world feels like too much, those two or three will feel like home.

How to Begin the Search

You don't need to go on a grand quest or attend countless social events. Often, your people come into view when you least expect it, in the most ordinary places—at a book club, during a yoga class, in a community garden, at your place of worship, or even online spaces built on real conversations, not clout.

Here are a few practical steps to help open the door:

1. **Get Clear on Your Values:** Know what matters to you. This will help you recognize when someone is aligned with your path.
2. **Engage in Activities That Reflect You:** Join groups or attend events that match your interests. This increases the chance of meeting like-hearted people.
3. **Show Up Authentically:** No need to over-share, but let people see the real you—your opinions, your humor, your honesty.
4. **Follow Energy, Not Image:** Pay attention to how you feel around people. Do you feel seen or drained? Respected or pressured? Choose based on how your body and spirit respond.
5. **Be Patient:** Deep connection takes time. Don't rush it. Let it build naturally.

Grieving the Ones Who Weren't Your People

Sometimes, finding your people means letting go of those who aren't. And that can hurt. Even toxic or mismatched relationships leave a void. It's okay to grieve them. It's okay to miss the memories or the hope you held for them.

But remember, peace is often the first sign that you're with the right people. If someone consistently disrupts your peace, no matter how long you've known them, it might be time to create distance.

Building a Safe Place to Land

When you do find your people, hold them gently. Tend to the relationship. Keep communication open. Respect their boundaries, as you want yours respected. Love them honestly, not perfectly.

You might:

- Schedule regular connection times.
- Send voice notes just to say you're thinking of them.
- Celebrate their little wins.
- Be the kind of friend you always needed.

Friendship, like any relationship, thrives when watered with time, attention, and truth.

Final Thoughts

You don't have to be everywhere or know everyone. You just need to find your circle—your safe place, your encouragers, your truth-tellers. In a loud, crowded world, that might be the bravest thing you ever do.

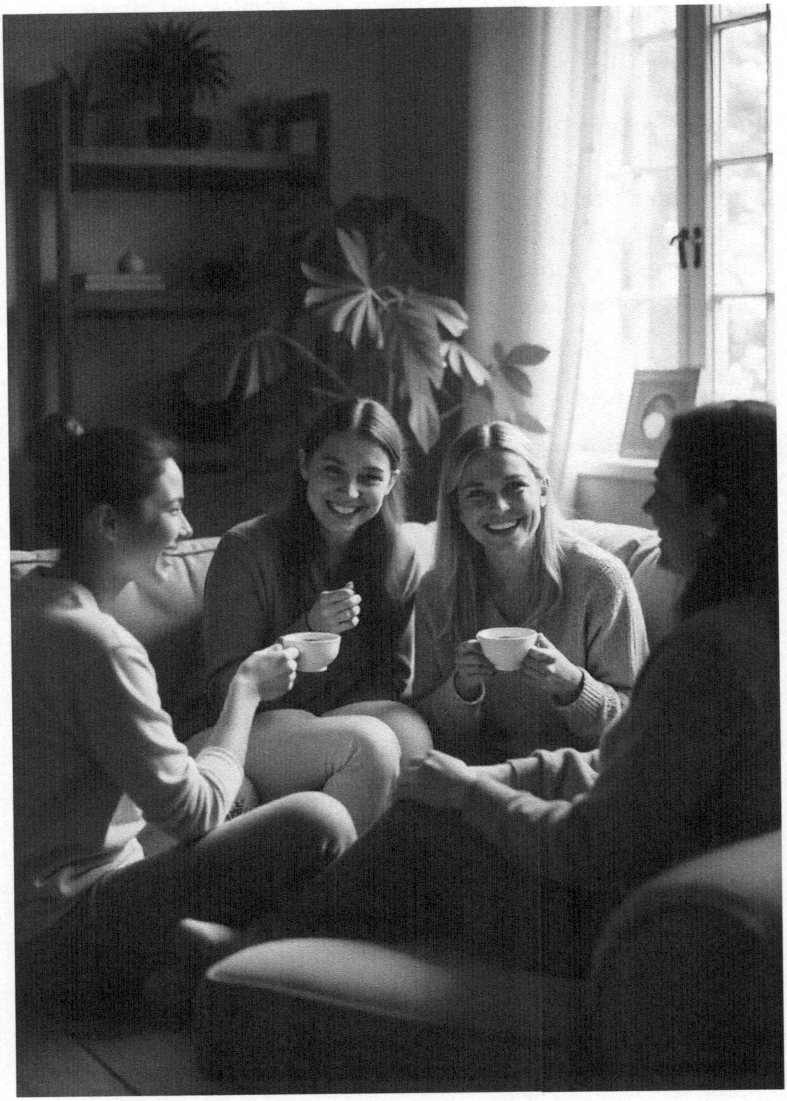

Section 6: Being Alone Without Feeling Lonely

In today's hyper-connected world, being alone can feel like a strange, almost taboo experience. We are constantly surrounded by the buzz of social media, group chats, office chatter, family responsibilities, and societal expectations to be social, productive, and available. But solitude isn't something to be feared—it's a sacred space, a restorative pause in the noise of the world. In this final section of Chapter 6, we'll explore the difference between loneliness and healthy solitude, and how learning to be alone can lead to deeper self-awareness, greater emotional resilience, and stronger relationships.

Understanding the Difference: Loneliness vs. Solitude

Let's begin by clearing a common misconception: being alone is not the same as being lonely. Loneliness is the distress we feel when we desire connection but don't have it. Solitude, on the other hand, is a choice to spend time with oneself—a quiet, comforting space that allows us to recharge and reconnect inwardly.

Imagine sitting by a lake at sunset with no one around. If your heart feels empty and yearning, that's loneliness. But if your heart feels full, calm, and grounded, you're in solitude. One is a wound; the other is a wellspring.

Too often, people avoid solitude because it triggers their insecurities. They fear the quiet, mistaking it for a void. But solitude isn't emptiness. It's presence—with yourself.

Why Solitude Is Essential for Emotional Health

When you allow yourself moments of solitude, you are tuning in to your inner world. You begin to hear your own voice—not the opinions of your friends, your boss, your family, or social media, but your authentic voice. This clarity helps you:

- Recognize your real desires.
- Set honest intentions.
- Develop creative ideas.
- Heal emotionally.
- Become a better communicator.

Without time alone, it's easy to become reactive, overcommitted, or emotionally burnt out. Solitude acts as a mirror. It helps you see your patterns clearly—the habits that serve you and those that don't.

The Fear of Being Alone

Many people resist being alone because they associate it with rejection or failure. Our culture often celebrates extroversion and constant busyness. When you choose solitude, others might misread it as isolation or antisocial behavior.

But being alone doesn't mean you lack love, friends, or meaning. In fact, people who enjoy solitude tend to have more emotionally fulfilling relationships because they're not clinging to others to complete them—they show up as whole.

If the idea of being alone scares you, ask yourself: what story am I telling myself about solitude? What discomfort is rising up, and what might it be trying to teach me?

Creating Meaningful Alone Time

Here are a few ways to intentionally invite solitude into your life and transform your relationship with being alone:

1. Design a solitude ritual: Pick a time each day—even if it's just 10 minutes—to be alone without distractions. No phone. No to-do lists. Just you. Light a candle, sip tea, take a walk, or simply sit and breathe.

2. Try solo dates: Take yourself out to lunch, visit a museum, or go on a solo hike. Bring a book, a journal, or just your thoughts. Notice how your mind behaves. Is it uncomfortable? Curious? Restless?

3. Embrace silence: Turn off the noise. Let yourself sit in the stillness without filling the air with music or chatter. What thoughts come up? What emotions rise? Greet them like old friends.

4. Practice self-dialogue: Write letters to yourself in a journal. Talk to yourself kindly. Reflect on your experiences without judgment. Ask: How am I, really?

5. Reframe the narrative: Instead of saying, "I'm alone," try saying, "I'm with myself." Language matters. It shapes how we experience reality.

How Solitude Strengthens Relationships

You might wonder: if solitude is so powerful, what does it have to do with healing relationships? Everything.

When you learn to enjoy your own company, you stop expecting others to fill your emotional gaps. That removes a huge burden from your relationships. You start showing up from a place of abundance rather than need.

You listen better. You judge less. You communicate more honestly. You set boundaries from a place of clarity.

Solitude also helps you notice who actually energizes you versus who drains you. You get clearer on your emotional bandwidth and what kind of connection you need in different seasons of life.

When Being Alone Turns Into Isolation

Of course, there's a line between nourishing solitude and unhealthy withdrawal. If you find yourself pulling away from everyone consistently, avoiding communication, or feeling numb or hopeless, that might be a sign of emotional overwhelm, depression, or burnout.

The key difference is intention. Solitude is chosen. Isolation often feels forced or reactive.

If you're unsure where you stand, reflect:

- Am I avoiding people out of fear or fatigue?
- Do I feel better or worse after being alone?
- Is my solitude energizing me or depleting me?

Seek support if you feel stuck. Therapists, coaches, or even honest conversations with trusted friends can help.

The Gift of Being Your Own Best Companion

When you cultivate the ability to be your own friend, your own comforter, and your own guide, you become emotionally sovereign. You carry your peace with you. Loneliness may still visit, but it doesn't rule you. You learn to hold space for it with compassion.

In solitude, you rediscover the sacred relationship with yourself—the one that grounds every other relationship you have.

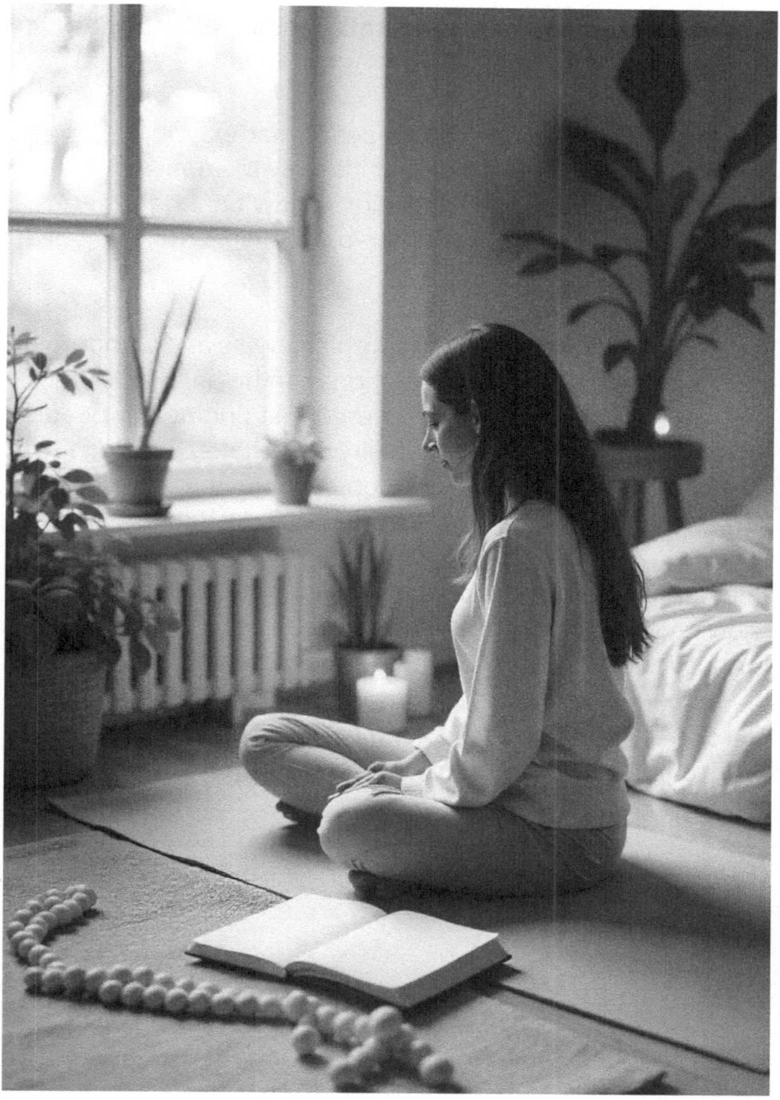

Chapter 6 Summary: Healing Relationships, Setting Boundaries

Chapter 6 reminded us that our peace matters more than pleasing others. We learned that it's okay to admit when people are draining, and we explored how boundaries are not walls but bridges to healthier, more respectful relationships.

We discussed how to set limits with kindness and without guilt, and how difficult conversations can be handled calmly and compassionately. We discovered that finding our people requires courage and intentionality, and that being alone isn't something to fear, but a sacred opportunity to connect with ourselves.

Ultimately, healing relationships begins within. It's about knowing your value, honoring your needs, and building connections that reflect your inner peace—not disrupt it.

You don't have to be available to everyone, and you don't have to fear being alone. You are already enough, exactly as you are.

Chapter 7: Building Your Personal Calm Toolkit
Section 1: Your Anxiety Warning Signals: How to Catch Them Early

Imagine this: you're sipping coffee, scrolling your phone, and suddenly your chest tightens. You can't quite explain why, but your heart is racing, your mind is spinning, and your stomach churns. That, right there, is anxiety knocking on your door.

But what if you could catch it before it barges in?

That's what this chapter is all about: building your *personal calm toolkit* by recognizing anxiety's early warning signs—before it escalates into a full-blown storm. Most people don't realize that anxiety gives you subtle whispers before it screams. If you can tune into those whispers, you can respond with self-compassion, boundaries, and tools to restore calm.

What Are Anxiety Warning Signals?

Think of anxiety as a highly sensitive alarm system. It's not the enemy. It's just trying to protect you. The problem is, it sometimes overreacts—like setting off the fire alarm when you burn toast.

Anxiety starts small. For one person, it might show up as jaw clenching. For another, it's procrastination. These are **signals**, not flaws.

Here are some of the most common early warning signs:

- **Physical**: racing heart, shallow breath, tension in neck or shoulders, digestive changes (like bloating, constipation, or nausea), sweaty palms.
- **Mental**: looping thoughts, difficulty focusing, catastrophizing, imagining worst-case scenarios.
- **Emotional**: irritability, edginess, a vague sense of dread, sudden overwhelm over small tasks.
- **Behavioral**: avoiding people or situations, snapping at loved ones, over-planning or control-seeking, mindless scrolling or snacking.

The moment you catch these signals, you've already begun the healing process. Awareness is your first tool.

Step One: Know Your Unique Signs

Everyone's anxiety is personalized. Just like allergies or food preferences, what stresses you out might not bother someone else.

Grab a journal (or your phone's notes app) and start noticing:

1. What happens in your body when you're anxious?
2. What thoughts or patterns repeat?
3. What behaviors follow?

For example:

- "My anxiety starts with a flutter in my chest, then I start checking emails obsessively."
- "I get snappy with my kids when I'm overwhelmed and then feel guilty."

This is not about judging yourself. It's about gently noticing patterns, like a compassionate detective.

Step Two: Track Your Triggers (Without Obsessing)

Once you've mapped out your signals, you can start seeing the patterns. Are there certain times of day, people, tasks, or even foods that consistently leave you feeling off-kilter?

Examples of triggers include:

- Crowded places
- Long to-do lists
- Lack of sleep
- Comparing yourself online
- Too much caffeine or sugar

Use this knowledge not to avoid life, but to *prepare* for it. Think of it like checking the weather forecast. If rain is coming, you don't cancel your day—you grab an umbrella.

Step Three: Create a Personalized Alert System

Once you know what your warning signs are, create your own calm code. This is a mental checklist or even a sticky note that says:

- "Pause. Breathe."
- "What is my body telling me right now?"
- "Have I had enough water, food, sleep?"
- "Do I need to step away for five minutes?"

You don't have to wait until you're in full panic mode. If your stomach twinges or you start biting your nails, that's your cue.

This is about learning to respond *early*, not reacting late.

Step Four: Build a Buffer Zone

A buffer zone is the emotional margin between you and the edge of burnout. Think of it as giving yourself space before you're forced to stop.

Ways to build a buffer:

- **Say no** before you're maxed out
- **Take five-minute breaks** between tasks
- **Check in with your body** every hour
- **Unplug** from digital noise
- **Go outside**, even briefly

These aren't luxuries. They're fuel stops for your nervous system.

Step Five: Share With Someone Safe

Sometimes we don't notice our anxiety until someone mirrors it back to us. Having one or two trusted people who know your early signals can be powerful.

You might say:

- "Hey, I tend to shut down when I'm overwhelmed. If you notice that, gently check in."

- "When I start canceling plans a lot, it might mean I'm too drained."

This isn't about depending on others to fix us. It's about inviting support into our healing process.

Step Six: Practice Micro-Calm Moments

Once you can catch anxiety early, you can meet it with micro-practices. These are tiny habits that interrupt the stress loop.

Examples:

- One-minute breathing
- Splashing cold water on your face
- Naming five things you can see and hear
- Putting your hand on your chest and saying, "I am safe."

These work best *before* the anxiety gets loud. Think of it like patching a small leak instead of waiting for a flood.

Why This Matters

Too often, we treat anxiety like an emergency room visit. We only notice it when it derails our lives. But imagine if we treated it like dental hygiene or hydration—a daily habit of checking in, noticing, and soothing ourselves.

This isn't about controlling your emotions. It's about learning the language of your nervous system so you can respond with grace instead of panic.

You deserve peace that starts *before* the breakdown.

Your Calm Toolkit Begins Here

This section lays the first stone in your personal calm toolkit. Just as a carpenter doesn't wait until a house is falling apart to grab a hammer, you don't have to wait for anxiety to break you down before you care for yourself.

Your early warning system is your first tool: the mirror that says, "Hey, something needs love."

Let's move forward and fill this toolkit with more tools, from grounding and breathwork to safe relationships and soul-nourishing habits.

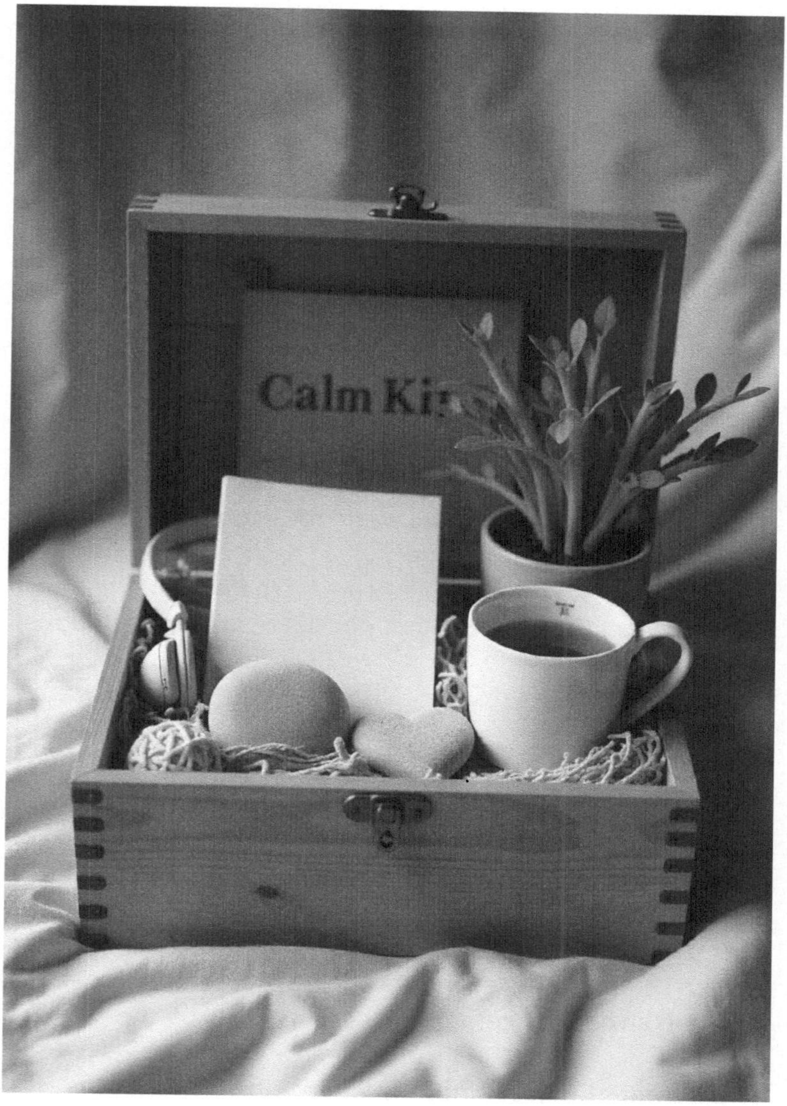
Calm Ki

Section 2: Creating Your "Calm Protocol" — A Custom Routine

If anxiety has taught us anything so far, it's this: there is no one-size-fits-all solution. What soothes your mind and body might not work for someone else, and that's not only okay—it's expected. This is why the concept of a "Calm Protocol" is not about rules or rigid habits. It's about building a toolkit and a routine you can trust. One that knows you. One that works with your lifestyle, your triggers, your rhythms.

Think of it as your personalized roadmap out of the fog. A clear set of steps you can follow when things feel overwhelming. When your chest tightens. When your thoughts speed up. When the world feels too loud.

In this section, we'll guide you through creating your very own Calm Protocol—a structure that doesn't restrict but supports.

What Is a Calm Protocol?

Imagine you're caught in a storm, and you have a sturdy backpack filled with exactly what you need to wait it out. A dry coat. A flashlight. A thermos of something warm. That's what your Calm Protocol is for emotional weather. It's your custom sequence of actions, tools, and practices you reach for when anxiety strikes.

It's different from just "knowing what helps." It's knowing **when to reach for what**, in what order, and how to make it easy to follow even when you're overwhelmed.

Let's build it step-by-step.

Step 1: Know Your Personal Signals

Before anything else, your Calm Protocol should begin with your warning signs. These are your body and mind's way of telling you, *"Hey, something's off."*

Use this prompt for a journaling exercise:

- Do your shoulders tense?
- Does your sleep get interrupted?
- Do you start avoiding people or tasks?
- Does your thinking get stuck in loops?

Write these down and label this part of your protocol as: **Recognize**.

Step 2: Identify What Actually Helps You Feel Grounded

Not what *should* help. What *does* help.

Go through your past experiences. Think about moments you felt yourself return to calm. What were you doing?

Maybe it was:

- Lying on the floor with your hand over your heart
- Stepping outside and looking at the sky
- Listening to a guided meditation
- Taking a hot shower
- Playing with your pet
- Moving your body (gently or vigorously)

List out at least 5 of these. These are your **calm anchors.**

Step 3: Pick Your "Immediate Reset" Tools

These are your go-to tools that work in under five minutes when you feel panic or overstimulation beginning to rise. This is the emergency first-aid kit.

Examples:

- Breathwork (Box breathing, 4-7-8 breathing)
- Splashing cold water on your face
- Tapping techniques (EFT)
- Holding a grounding object (stone, sensory toy, textured item)

Pick two to three that feel **accessible** in any situation. This becomes your **Reset** section.

Step 4: Define Your "Regulate" Routine

Once the immediate storm passes, we move to regulation. This isn't about fixing everything instantly. It's about gradually calming your nervous system and reminding your body: *You're safe now.*

This part of the protocol includes:

- A soothing playlist
- Gentle stretches or a short walk
- A nourishing snack or warm drink
- A 10-minute journaling session

You can choose to set this up in a way that suits your life—morning, evening, or even lunchtime. The key is consistency. Think of this as your nervous system's daily vitamin.

Step 5: Schedule in Preventative Care

Your protocol isn't only for when you're overwhelmed. It's also about building resilience. Include practices that *strengthen* your ability to handle future stress.

These might include:

- Weekly check-in with yourself (journal, walk, prayer, therapy)
- Monthly social detox
- Quiet solo time doing something creative
- Limiting news or social media after 8 p.m.

This step is called **Restore**.

Step 6: Put It All Together (With Flexibility!)

Now let's combine everything into a simple framework:

Your Calm Protocol:

1. **Recognize** – Early signs of anxiety
2. **Reset** – Immediate tools (breathing, grounding)
3. **Regulate** – Calming activities after the spike
4. **Restore** – Ongoing practices to prevent burnout

You can write this down on an index card, create a voice memo for yourself, or use a notes app on your phone. Make it accessible, visible, and **non-judgmental.**

This is not a performance. This is a promise to your nervous system: "When you ring the alarm, I'll listen. And I know what to do."

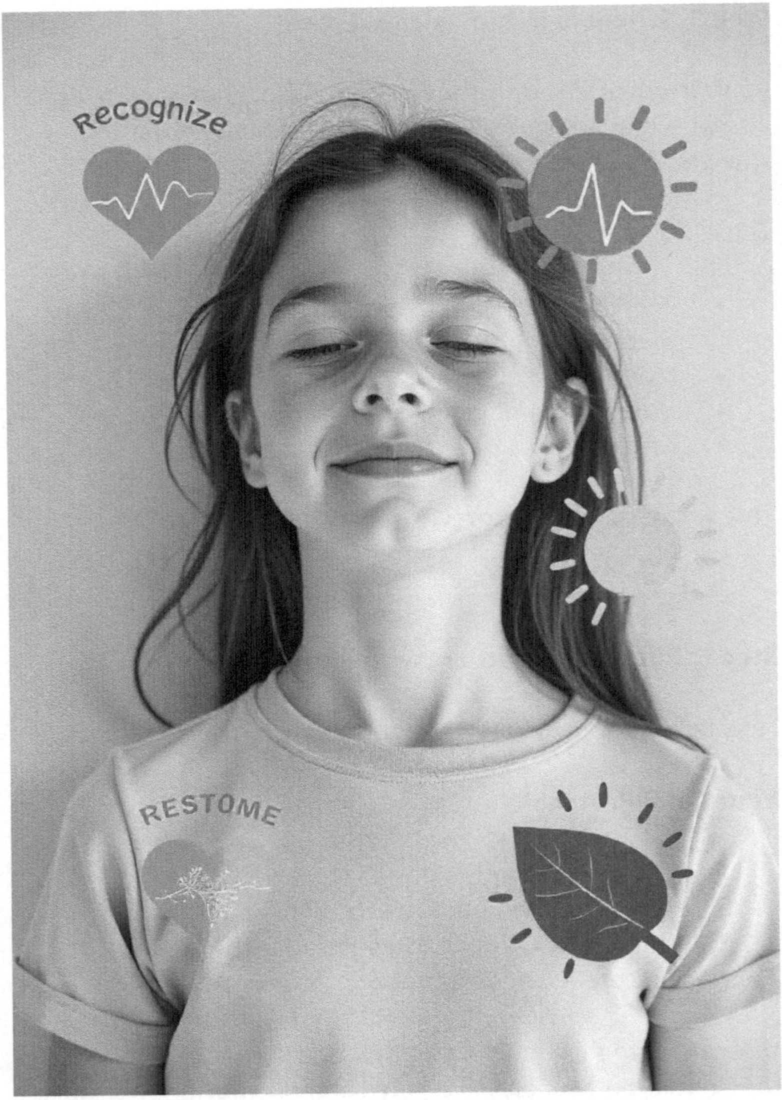
Recognize
RESTOME

A Note on Personality Types and Customizing Further

Your Calm Protocol should be a reflection of **you.** If you're a highly sensitive person (HSP), your toolkit might emphasize nature, texture, and quiet. If you're more extroverted, your calm might come from movement, voice notes, or calling a friend.

Give yourself permission to adapt it as you grow. Your needs today may not be your needs six months from now.

What If It Doesn't Work One Day?

That's okay. Protocols are not perfection. Sometimes the storm is stronger than the plan. But having a structure—even if it's not perfect—reminds you that you are not powerless. You are not starting from zero every time.

The key is not in how flawlessly you follow it, but that you **remember to turn to it.**

Final Reflection: Your Calm Is Learnable

We often think calm is something you either have or don't. But it's not innate. It's learnable. And building your Calm Protocol is a powerful act of self-trust. You're teaching yourself how to self-regulate, how to honor your needs, and how to return to your center—again and again.

So take your time. Revisit it monthly. Update it after tough weeks. Treat it like a living document.

This is not about being unshakable. It's about being able to find your footing again, no matter what life throws at you.

Section 3: Emotional First-Aid for Overwhelming Days

There are days when everything feels like too much. Your to-do list is a mile long. A conversation from the morning is still echoing in your mind. You spilled coffee, forgot a password, missed a call—and somehow, all of it feels like proof that you're not doing okay.

Welcome to an overwhelming day. We all have them. And when they strike, they can leave us feeling powerless and emotionally raw. That's why it's important to build what I like to call an "Emotional First-Aid Kit."

This isn't a metaphorical idea. It's a real, tangible, go-to plan you design ahead of time so that when everything feels like it's falling apart, you know exactly what to reach for—emotionally, mentally, and physically.

Why You Need an Emotional First-Aid Kit

When we're emotionally overwhelmed, our nervous system enters a stress response: fight, flight, freeze, or fawn. This isn't a time when you can think clearly, make good decisions, or recall your favorite grounding technique from three weeks ago.

Having a personal protocol prepared ahead of time is like packing an umbrella before the storm. It's a form of radical self-care—not just about survival, but about learning to thrive even on the hardest days.

What Goes in Your Emotional First-Aid Kit?

Everyone's kit will look different, and that's the beauty of it. The goal is to assemble tools, reminders, and strategies that help you stabilize your emotions, reconnect with yourself, and regulate your nervous system.

1. A Safe Space

Identify a physical or mental space where you feel safe and secure. This could be a corner of your room with a cozy blanket, a park bench under your favorite tree, or even a visualization you close your eyes and return to when things get hard.

2. Comfort Items

Include items that soothe your senses:

- A soft scarf or piece of fabric
- Essential oils or scented candles (lavender, eucalyptus, or sandalwood)
- A playlist of calming music
- A comforting photo or token

These tactile or sensory items help bring you back to the present moment.

3. Breath and Body Tools

Include 1-2 techniques you can practice easily:

- Box breathing (Inhale 4 counts, hold 4, exhale 4, hold 4)
- Legs-up-the-wall pose
- Self-hug or tapping (EFT)

Remember: Your body is the bridge back to calm. These tools help you cross it.

4. Words That Ground You

Overwhelming days distort our thoughts. Having a written note to yourself can remind you of the truth:

"I've survived every hard day before this one. I can survive this too."

"My feelings are valid, but they are not forever."

Write 2-3 personal affirmations or encouragements in your own handwriting. Keep them where you can read them.

5. Emergency Journal Prompt

Write down a go-to journaling prompt like:

- "Right now, I feel..."
- "What do I need most in this moment?"
- "What is one thing I can do to soothe myself today?"

You don't need to write a novel. Even a few lines can help you emotionally exhale.

6. A Grounding Object or Ritual

Choose one small object to carry with you: a stone, a cross, a small piece of wood, or a shell. Touch it when you feel overwhelmed. Let it anchor you. Or choose a ritual like making tea, washing your face, or lighting a candle as a moment to pause and begin again.

How to Use Your Kit

Think of your Emotional First-Aid Kit as your reset button.

When the overwhelm hits:

1. **Notice the signs:** Are you short-tempered? Teary? Overreacting? Shutting down? This is your signal.
2. **Pause without judgment:** Don't ask yourself why you feel this way. Ask yourself: *What can I do right now to care for me?*
3. **Use one tool:** You don't need the whole kit. Just start with one small step—put on your calming music, hold your grounding object, or read your affirmation.
4. **Come back to yourself:** As the wave passes, gently return to the moment. Don't rush the reset. Give yourself grace.

Creating a Visible Ritual

The power of the Emotional First-Aid Kit comes not only from having it but from *using* it consistently. Create a visual reminder for your kit:

- A small box or pouch with your tools in it
- A note on your phone with your steps
- A photo collage of your safe space
- A dedicated drawer or bag you can reach for

You are training your brain to understand: "When I feel overwhelmed, I know what to do."

The Role of Compassion

There will be days when even your emotional toolkit doesn't seem to "work."

And that's okay.

This isn't about fixing yourself. It's about meeting yourself in the hard moments with gentleness.

Sometimes your best first-aid is simply sitting still and saying:

"This is hard. And I am doing the best I can."

Because you are. You always have been.

Real-Life Example: Anna's First-Aid Ritual

Anna is a single mom who works remotely and cares for her aging parent. Overwhelming days are not the exception—they're the norm. She used to numb her feelings with food and late-night scrolling. Then, she created her Emotional First-Aid Kit.

Now, when the panic rises, Anna lights a lavender candle, steps outside to breathe for two minutes, and writes in a notebook where she tracks her emotional highs and lows. It's not perfect, but it's consistent. And she says, "It's like telling myself, 'I see you. I've got you.'"

That's the power of this ritual. It's not about changing your life overnight. It's about reminding yourself you are not alone in your life.

Reflection Prompt

Take a moment to journal:

- What do your overwhelming days usually look like?
- Which tool above speaks to you the most?
- What would you include in your emotional first-aid kit?

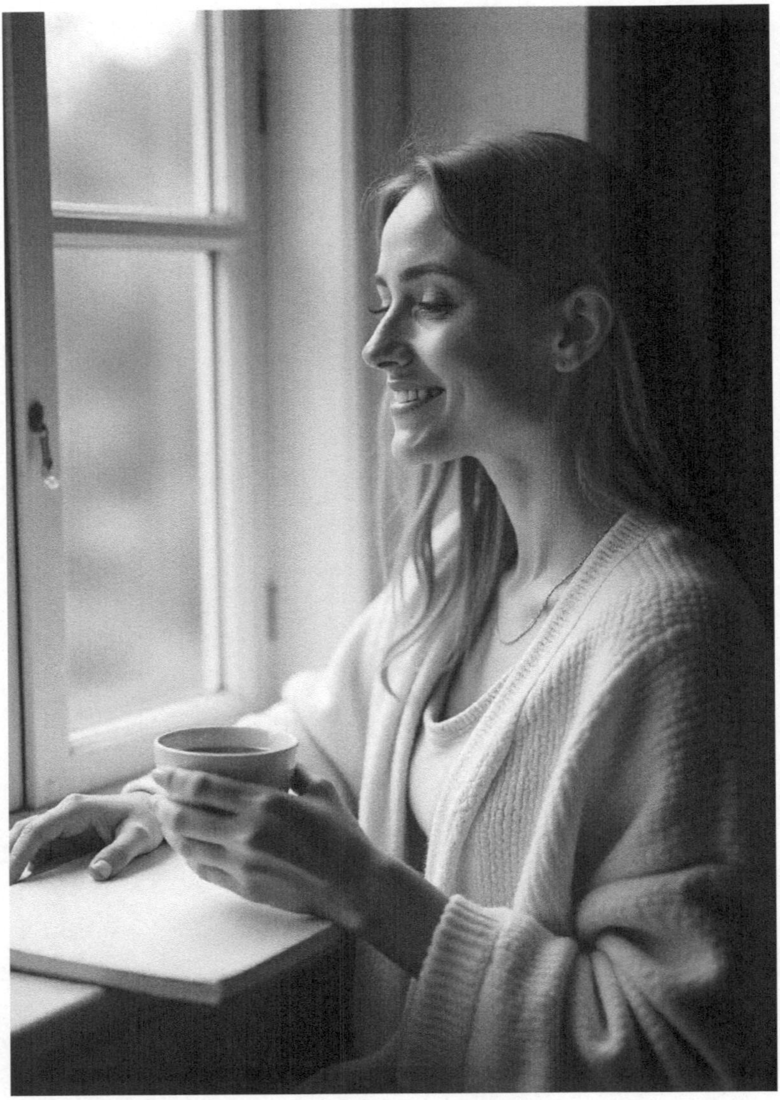

Section 4: Habits That Stick (and How to Build Them)

By now, you've built a solid foundation in understanding your anxiety triggers, crafted a personalized calm protocol, and learned strategies to manage overwhelming days. But even the best plan can falter without consistent habits that support it. In this section, we focus on turning your calm practices into daily habits — habits that stick, not just for a week or two, but for a lifetime.

Why Most Habits Fail (and Why That's Okay)

We often approach habits with all-or-nothing thinking: either we do them perfectly every day, or we fail. This mindset sets us up for disappointment. Real, lasting habits aren't born from perfection. They're born from repetition, grace, and realistic expectations.

A 2010 study from University College London found it takes, on average, 66 days to form a habit — not the 21 days we often hear. And that's an average. Some habits can take over 200 days to stick. So if you've struggled to maintain change before, it doesn't mean you're weak — it means you're human.

The good news? Every step counts. Every attempt lays groundwork. And with the right tools, you can make your peace-centered habits automatic.

Step 1: Start Smaller Than You Think You Should

When it comes to building a new habit, we often start too big. "I'll meditate for 30 minutes every day." "I'll journal every night before bed." "I'll walk for an hour each morning."

Instead, ask yourself: *What is the smallest, most laughably easy version of this habit I can do daily?* That's where success begins.

- Instead of 30 minutes of meditation, commit to 3 minutes.
- Instead of journaling a full page, commit to one sentence.
- Instead of a 60-minute walk, start with 5 minutes outside.

You're not lowering the bar to cheat yourself. You're building momentum. And momentum is more important than intensity in the beginning.

Step 2: Link the Habit to an Existing Routine

One of the most powerful strategies is **habit stacking** — pairing a new habit with something you already do daily. This gives your brain a cue to follow and creates a natural rhythm.

Examples:

- After brushing your teeth in the morning, breathe deeply for one minute.
- After pouring your coffee, write one gratitude sentence in your journal.
- Before turning off the bedroom light, stretch your arms for 30 seconds.

When the new habit is attached to a familiar action, it becomes anchored — and much harder to forget.

Step 3: Make It Visible and Attractive

Your environment is the silent partner in every habit you form. If your calming habits are hidden — your journal in a drawer, your yoga mat in the closet — you're far less likely to engage with them.

Design your environment for ease:

- Place your journal on your pillow each morning.
- Keep your water bottle on your desk as a visual reminder to hydrate.
- Use a sticky note with a calming affirmation on your bathroom mirror.

Visual cues trigger action. The more visible and inviting the habit, the more it calls you to engage.

Step 4: Track the Habit (But Gently)

Habit tracking doesn't need to be complicated. A simple checkmark on a calendar or a habit app can create a sense of satisfaction and momentum.

Why it works:

- It gives your brain a reward.
- It creates a visual chain — and most people don't like breaking a chain once they start.
- It builds accountability, even if only to yourself.

Important: Be gentle with yourself. If you miss a day, it's not a failure. It's a pause. Consistency over time is the goal — not perfection.

Step 5: Revisit and Evolve Your Habits Regularly

What serves you today might not serve you six months from now. Check in with your calm routine monthly or quarterly. Ask yourself:

- Is this habit still helping me?
- Has it become automatic?
- Do I need to shift it, stretch it, or simplify it?

Your life changes — and your habits should evolve with it.

Habit Formula Recap

Here's a simple 5-step habit-building formula you can apply to any calming practice:

1. **Anchor it** to something you already do.
2. **Make it easy** — start laughably small.
3. **Make it visible** — design your space to remind you.
4. **Track it** — celebrate consistency, not perfection.
5. **Revisit it** — evolve as needed.

Real-Life Examples: Habits That Stick

Let's look at a few examples from real people building habits that support inner calm:

Nora, 41, marketing consultant
Habit: Breathing pause

- Anchored to: First email check in the morning

- Tiny version: 3 slow breaths before opening her inbox
- Result: "It puts me in control instead of reacting to chaos."

Adil, 28, grad student
Habit: Body scan meditation

- Anchored to: Getting into bed at night
- Tiny version: 30 seconds of breath awareness
- Result: "It helps me sleep better and feel less wired."

Grace, 34, single mom
Habit: Gratitude journaling

- Anchored to: Dinner clean-up
- Tiny version: One sentence per night
- Result: "Even on hard days, I see something good."

When a Habit Slips — And It Will

You will forget. You will skip days. Life will interrupt you.

Here's the rule: *Never miss twice.* One miss is human. Two in a row starts a pattern.

If you do miss two or more days, don't start with shame. Restart with the smallest version of the habit again.

Remember: it's not about streaks. It's about building a life where calm shows up often, without effort.

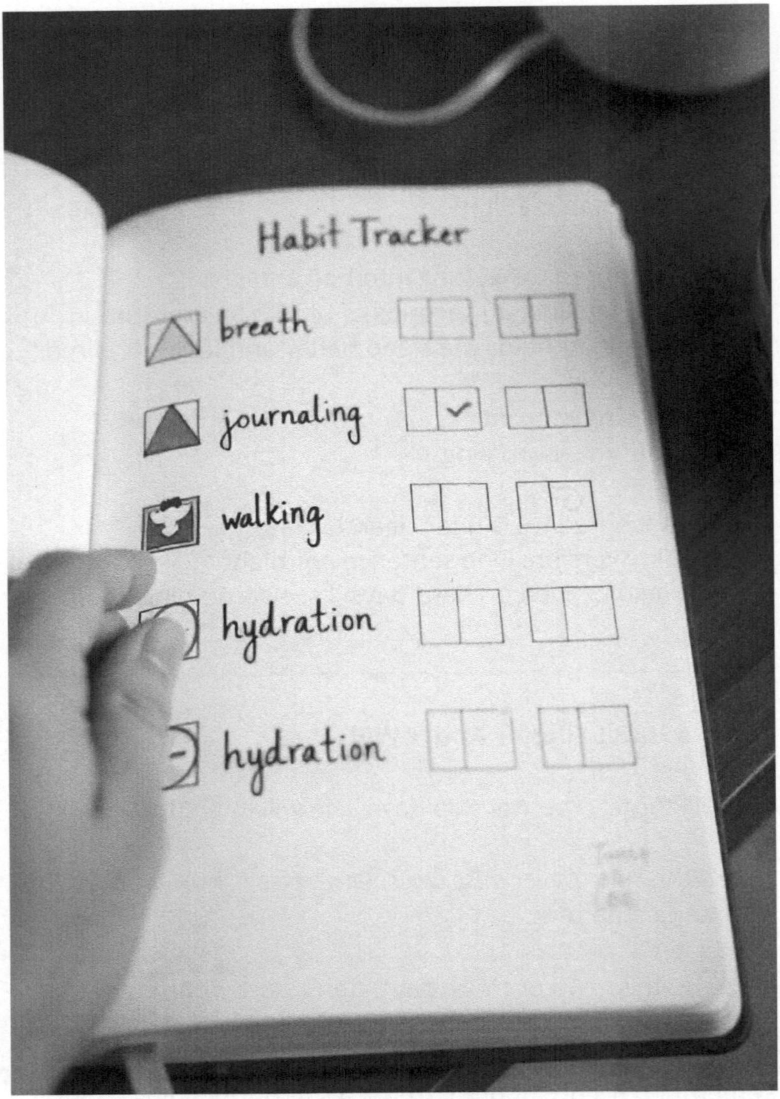
Habit Tracker
breath
journaling
walking
hydration
hydration

Integrating Habits into Your Calm Toolkit

Each habit you build becomes a **tool** in your personal calm toolkit. The goal isn't to do all of them every day, but to have them available when life gets loud.

You don't need a dozen habits to feel calm — just a few that matter. Ones that fit your life. Ones that feel like a gift, not a task.

Section 5: Learning to Reset, Not Quit

Have you ever had a day when everything felt off track? You missed your morning routine, forgot an important task, argued with a loved one, or just felt heavy and unmotivated. And then came that voice in your head: "Well, that's it. I've failed. Might as well give up."

Let's challenge that voice.

Learning to reset—not quit—is one of the most powerful tools in your calm toolkit. This is the mindset shift that transforms temporary slips into opportunities for resilience. Life doesn't reward perfection. It rewards those who keep showing up, even when things don't go as planned.

What Does "Reset" Really Mean?

A reset is a gentle pause, a conscious choice to realign without judgment. It's not about punishment, shame, or over-correction. Instead, it's about stepping out of the downward spiral before it gains momentum.

Imagine pressing a "soft reboot" on your day. You're not erasing everything—you're simply starting from where you are, with kindness.

A reset might look like:

- Taking three deep breaths before the next meeting.
- Closing your eyes for five minutes of stillness.
- Writing down one thing you're grateful for.
- Drinking a glass of water.
- Apologizing, then letting go.

These may seem small, but they are powerful cues to your nervous system that you're choosing calm over chaos.

Why Quitting Feels Easier

Quitting gives us an illusion of control. When things feel overwhelming or imperfect, quitting offers a way out of the discomfort. But that "relief" is often temporary.

We quit because:

- We believe one bad moment defines everything.
- We fear starting over.
- We're chasing perfection instead of consistency.
- We're tired—not of the habit, but of being hard on ourselves.

Here's the truth: it's not about never falling—it's about getting better at standing back up, without shame. That's what growth looks like.

Micro-Resets Throughout the Day

You don't need to wait until tomorrow to begin again. Micro-resets are like emotional pit-stops—quick refuels for your mental energy.

Examples of micro-resets:

- **1-minute reset:** Step outside, breathe fresh air, feel the ground beneath you.
- **5-minute reset:** Brew a cup of tea, journal a few lines, or stretch gently.
- **10-minute reset:** Take a mindful walk without your phone, wash your face, or meditate.

These resets don't require grand effort. They simply invite you back to the present.

The Power of Grace-Based Living

We often think grit is what builds habits. But what if grace is even more powerful?

Grace is the voice that says:

- "You didn't fail—you're human."
- "Today was hard. That doesn't mean tomorrow will be."
- "Let's begin again."

When you combine grit (the willingness to try) with grace (the willingness to forgive), you become unstoppable.

You stop fearing failure because you know how to reset.

You stop chasing perfection because you've discovered progress.

You stop giving up on yourself because you've learned how to start again.

Your Reset Ritual: A Personal Formula

Let's create a simple Reset Ritual that works for you.

Use this 3-step framework:

1. Recognize the Need:
Catch the warning signals. Are you:

- Feeling scattered or snappy?
- Criticizing yourself constantly?
- Procrastinating or avoiding?

These are signs you need a reset, not a lecture.

2. Pause + Breathe:
Even 60 seconds of intentional breathing can shift your internal state. Try the 4-7-8 method:

- Inhale for 4 counts
- Hold for 7 counts
- Exhale for 8 counts

Do this 3–4 times. That's it.

3. Reconnect with Calm:
Ask yourself: "What would support me right now?"

- A walk?
- A text to a friend?
- A nourishing snack?
- A playlist that shifts your energy?

The key is to make your reset actionable and compassionate.

What If You Miss a Week?

Let's address the fear head-on.

Maybe you started journaling daily, meditating, or waking up earlier—and then life happened. The routine fell apart. A part of you wonders, "Did I just waste all that effort?"

No.

Progress doesn't vanish because of a pause. Habits live in the *return*, not the streak. Every time you return, you reinforce the belief: *I am someone who chooses calm.*

This builds identity-based habits—the kind that last.

So instead of, "I failed," try:
"I'm resetting. Because I matter."

Encouragement for the Road

You are not behind. You are not broken. You don't need to earn rest.

You're allowed to reset as many times as you need. That's not weakness—it's resilience.

Some days will be smooth. Others will be jagged. But you carry within you the tools to begin again, and again, and again.

That's your superpower.

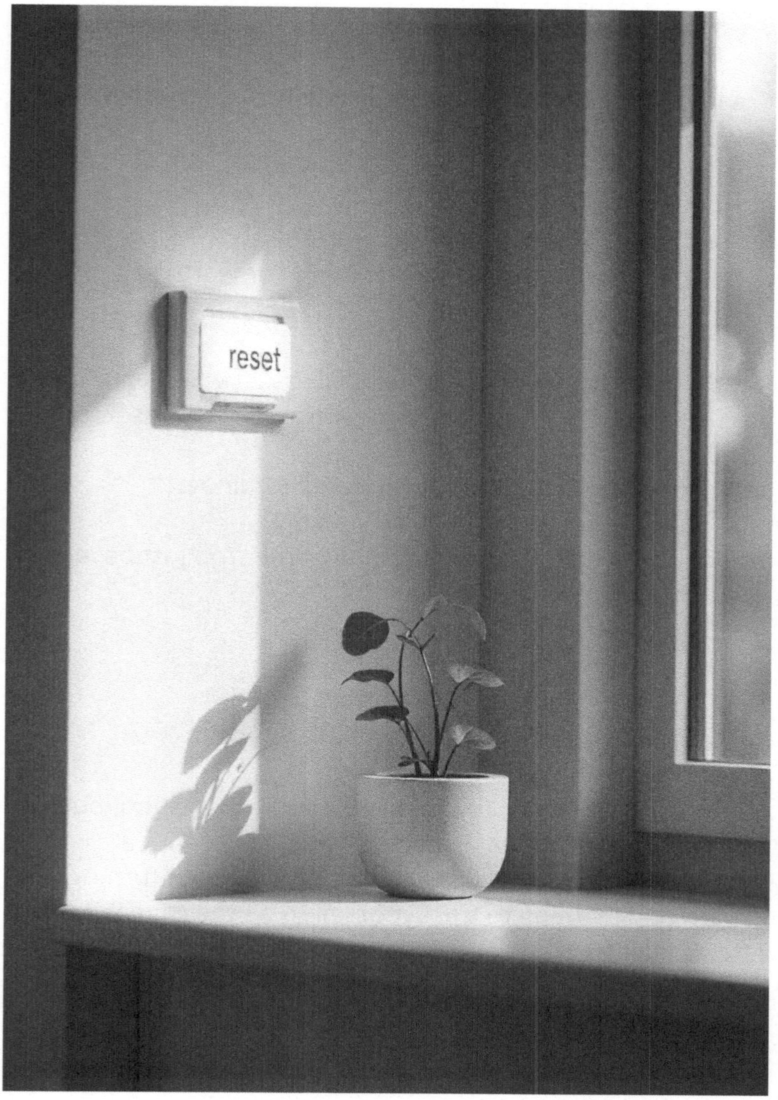
reset

Try This Today: Your Reset Card

Create a small card or note titled: **"My Reset Ritual"** Write down:

- 3 signs you need a reset
- 3 micro-actions that calm you
- A mantra that reminds you of your worth (e.g., "I can begin again.")

Keep it in your bag, wallet, or journal. Use it when your mind says, "Just give up." Instead, you'll whisper, "Let's reset."

Let's close this section with a powerful reminder:

You don't have to finish strong every time. You just have to keep showing up—with grace.

And that is more than enough.

Section 6: Becoming Your Own Safe Space

In a world that moves too fast and often expects too much, becoming your own safe space is not a luxury—it's a necessity. This final section of Chapter 7 is about turning inward and learning to trust yourself to be the calm you seek. After building awareness, designing calm protocols, managing emotional first-aid, developing habits, and learning to reset instead of quit, it all comes together in one powerful truth: your deepest peace comes from within.

The Concept of a Safe Space Within

A safe space is often defined as a physical place—a cozy corner, a quiet room, a retreat in nature. But what if your safest place could be you? Imagine being able to come home to yourself, no matter where you are. You wouldn't have to rely on external circumstances to feel okay. Your thoughts, your breath, your presence could be the place you go to when life feels chaotic.

Becoming your own safe space means:

- Responding to anxiety with compassion instead of judgment.
- Holding space for your emotions without needing to fix or suppress them.
- Cultivating a consistent practice of inner stillness, even when the outer world is noisy.

This practice isn't about perfection. It's about presence.

Why We Struggle to Feel Safe with Ourselves

Let's be honest: many of us are far more comfortable taking care of others than being alone with ourselves. That discomfort is often rooted in past experiences—childhood moments where emotions were dismissed, trauma that taught us not to trust our instincts, or a world that rewarded constant output and performance over rest and reflection.

Sometimes, the noise inside our heads feels louder than the world outside. Thoughts like:

- "You're not doing enough."
- "Why do you feel this way again?"
- "You should be stronger than this."

These internal narratives can create a hostile environment in our own minds. If our inner voice constantly criticizes or pressures us, of course we don't feel safe within ourselves.

But you can change that. You can rewire your internal environment with gentle consistency, the way you'd create a warm home one soft touch at a time.

Ways to Become Your Own Safe Space

1. Develop a Daily Self-Check-In

Ask yourself:

- How am I feeling right now?
- What do I need?
- What would be the most loving thing I could offer myself in this moment?

This doesn't need to be a long process. Even two mindful minutes in the morning or evening can be enough. The goal isn't to solve anything—just to acknowledge your inner landscape.

2. Create Inner Boundaries

Inner boundaries are just as important as outer ones. These are the mental limits you set with yourself for the sake of emotional safety:

- Choosing not to spiral into overthinking by practicing presence.
- Refusing to believe every negative thought that arises.
- Limiting exposure to negative inner dialogues.

A simple mantra like, "This thought is not the truth" can act as an inner boundary line when your mind goes into overdrive.

3. Have a Reassurance Ritual

Create a calming ritual that reminds you of your inner strength. This could be:

- Placing a hand over your heart and repeating a truth like, "I am safe now."
- Reading a passage from a book that grounds you.
- Listening to a calming playlist that feels like an emotional reset.

Let your body and brain associate these acts with safety.

4. Practice Self-Compassionate Talk

Instead of reacting with criticism when you're anxious or overwhelmed, practice saying:

- "Of course you're feeling this way. It makes sense."
- "I'm here for you. I'm listening."
- "Let's take this one step at a time."

These phrases, spoken gently, signal to your nervous system that it doesn't need to stay in fight-or-flight mode.

5. Return to the Breath

Your breath is a built-in tool for self-regulation. Practice pausing in moments of stress to take three slow, conscious breaths. Let each inhale be a reminder of your strength and each exhale a release of tension.

Over time, this becomes a habit. Your breath becomes your anchor.

You Are the Calm You're Searching For

One of the greatest illusions of modern life is that peace is something we have to chase. It's always just one achievement away, one vacation away, one relationship or resolution away. But real calm isn't a place. It's a presence—and it's yours to build.

In becoming your own safe space, you:

- Trust your capacity to soothe yourself.
- Know how to pause without giving up.
- Develop a toolkit that honors your real-life challenges and your quiet strength.

Summary of Chapter 7: Building Your Personal Calm Toolkit

Chapter 7 brought all the tools of this journey together and gave you a blueprint to return to again and again:

1. **Your Anxiety Warning Signals:** You learned how to identify the earliest signs of stress before they explode. Tuning into your body's signals helps you respond early and gently.
2. **Your Calm Protocol:** You designed (or started designing) a custom routine that works for you. This protocol isn't rigid—it's responsive. It's what you reach for when life feels too much.
3. **Emotional First-Aid:** You were given a set of immediate practices to ground and reframe on overwhelming days. These are practical, compassionate, and flexible.
4. **Habits That Stick:** We explored how real change is built slowly and with care. You saw how to start small

and stay steady, choosing systems over sudden motivation.

5. **Learning to Reset, Not Quit:** This section empowered you to see that off days don't cancel your progress. They're invitations to return with grace, not reasons to abandon the journey.
6. **Becoming Your Own Safe Space:** Finally, you learned the value of turning inward. You are not broken or behind. You are becoming your own refuge, your own calm.

This is not about never feeling anxious again. It's about knowing what to do when anxiety shows up. It's about building a life that gently supports you.

You now have the tools. You now have the awareness. And most importantly, you now know that peace is possible—and it starts with you.

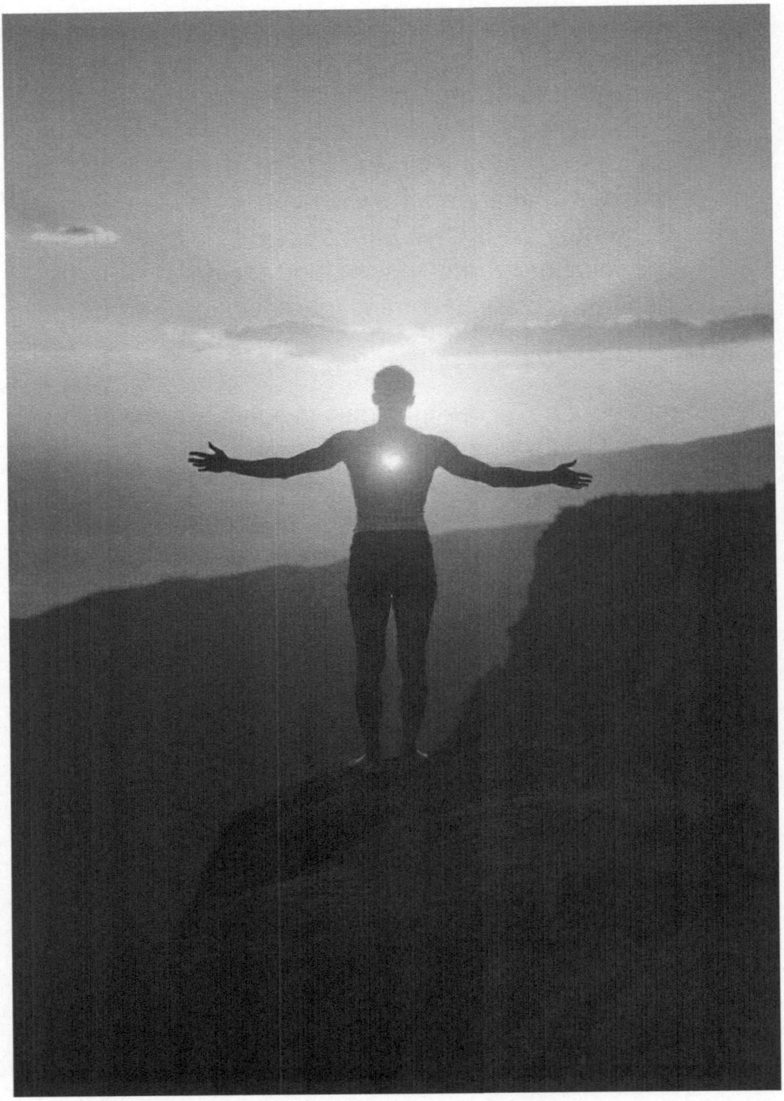

Chapter 8: The Long Game — Living With Resilience and Hope

Section 1: What Long-Term Calm Really Looks Like

Peace isn't a final destination, a prize you win at the end of some grueling mental marathon. It's not the quiet after the storm, or a once-in-a-lifetime vacation that makes your soul sigh in relief. Peace, when you really get to know it, is something more subtle, more lived-in. It's a rhythm, a tone that underlies the highs and lows of life. This chapter is about building that rhythm for the long haul — not a moment of escape, but a lifestyle of grounded calm and steady hope.

The Illusion of Arrival

Most of us grow up thinking that calm is something we get once everything else is in order. We tell ourselves, *"I'll feel peaceful when I have enough money, when I find the right relationship, when I lose the weight, when work is less stressful."* But here's the truth that life keeps trying to teach us: peace doesn't wait for your circumstances to be perfect.

Long-term calm is not about the absence of stress. It's about how you meet that stress. It's about learning to breathe even when the air feels tight. It's about cultivating internal tools that remind you: *You are okay, even when everything else isn't.*

Think of calm like a home you carry inside yourself. Some days, the world will knock on your door loudly. But when your foundation is strong, you don't crumble. You sit with the noise, knowing it will pass. You light a candle anyway.

Resilience: The Quiet Companion of Calm

Many people associate calm with being passive, laid-back, or emotionless. But calm is not a lack of passion or engagement. It is **deep resilience**. It is the ability to keep showing up without being swallowed by the tide.

Resilience is:

- Answering emails even when anxiety tells you to hide.
- Saying "no" even when guilt comes knocking.
- Letting go of what you can't control without giving up on what you can.

And here's the twist: **Resilience and calm feed each other**. The more resilient you become, the calmer you feel because you trust yourself. You know you can face what comes.

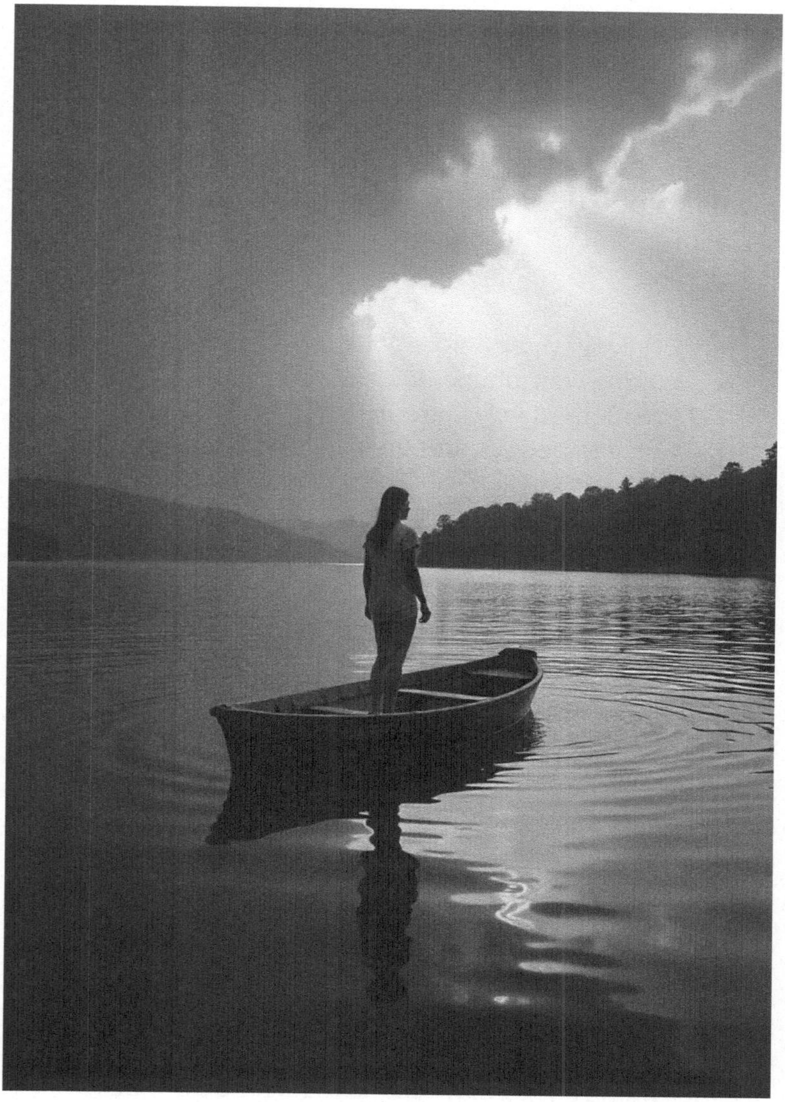

Tiny Moments, Big Impact

When we imagine calm, we often think of grand gestures — quitting your job, moving to a quiet village, meditating on a mountain. But real, long-term calm comes from **tiny moments practiced consistently**.

It looks like:

- Drinking water before your coffee.
- Putting your phone down during meals.
- Breathing slowly in traffic.
- Going to bed without finishing the to-do list.

These small actions teach your nervous system that you are safe. Over time, they build a relationship of trust with your body and mind.

Long-term calm is cumulative. Every little choice matters.

Adapting Your Calm to Life Seasons

Let's be real: life doesn't stay the same. Kids grow up, jobs change, losses come, and new dreams arrive. That's why it's important not to tie your calm to a strict routine or a specific method.

Instead, build a toolkit of practices that can shift with your seasons:

- When you're busy, your calm might be five deep breaths in the bathroom.
- When you're grieving, your calm might be silence and solitude.
- When you're joyful, your calm might be savoring it without fear.

Your long-term calm should feel flexible, not rigid. It's a friend that walks beside you, not a rule that controls you.

Reframing Progress

You will still have anxious days. You will still snap, overthink, and spiral from time to time. That doesn't mean you've lost your calm. It means you're human.

Progress in the long game looks like:

- Bouncing back faster.
- Recognizing your patterns.
- Speaking to yourself with more kindness.
- Asking for help when you need it.

Give yourself permission to be **a work in progress with peace in your pocket**.

Hope as a Calm Strategy

Hope isn't just a nice idea. It's a strategy. It fuels long-term calm because it gives your nervous system a reason to **not panic**. When you believe tomorrow can be better, you breathe easier today.

But hope is not naive optimism. It's not ignoring the hard stuff. Hope says:

- *"This is tough, but it won't last forever."*
- *"I've made it through before; I can again."*
- *"There are still good things coming."*

Quote Box: *"Hope is the quiet courage that keeps lighting the candle, even when the power's out."*

Building a Lifestyle, Not a Crisis Response

In previous chapters, we explored how to calm your mind in the moment. But now, it's time to zoom out.

Ask yourself:

- What kind of calm do I want to live with?
- What do I want my daily life to *feel* like?
- Who helps me feel grounded?
- What choices restore me?

Long-term peace is about alignment. Not perfection, not performance. Just a way of life that feels honest, gentle, and strong.

That might mean less noise. That might mean more boundaries. That might mean becoming okay with missing out.

And all of that is worth it.

Reflection Questions

1. What does peace look like in my life right now?
2. What daily habits help me feel calm and centered?
3. What old beliefs keep pulling me away from long-term calm?
4. What new definition of peace am I ready to accept?

Section 2: Dealing With Setbacks and Emotional Triggers

Setbacks are not just detours; they are part of the road. And emotional triggers? They are the rumble strips on that road—warning signs asking us to slow down, pay attention, and take care. Learning to deal with them doesn't mean eliminating them. It means understanding them, working with them, and building strategies to bounce back instead of breaking down.

When life feels like it's unraveling, when old wounds reopen with just a word or a glance, when progress feels erased by one mistake—that's when our real work begins. Not the glamorous, Instagram-worthy version of healing, but the gritty, quiet, unseen work of resilience.

What a Setback Really Means

A setback isn't a sign that you're failing. It's a signal that you're still learning. Growth isn't linear; it looks more like a tangled ball of yarn than a straight upward arrow. Some days you leap forward. Some days you slide back. Both are part of the same journey.

Maybe your anxiety flares up again after weeks of calm. Maybe an old habit reappears when you're stressed. Maybe a single comment makes you feel like the person you used to be—the one you've worked so hard to outgrow. It's tempting in those moments to feel like you're back at square one. But you're not. The fact that you notice it, that you're aware of what's happening, that you care about how far you've come—that's growth.

Understanding Emotional Triggers

Emotional triggers are not your enemies. They are messengers. They show you where you're still healing. Think of them as emotional bruises—you don't realize how tender something is until it gets touched. That doesn't mean you're weak. It means you're human.

A trigger might be a tone of voice, a certain look, a smell, a location, a time of year. It might come out of nowhere and hit you in the middle of an otherwise normal day. Instead of reacting with shame, try responding with curiosity:

- Why did this affect me so strongly?
- What memory or belief is this connected to?
- What do I need right now to feel safe again?

This is the inner dialogue that helps you turn emotional reactivity into emotional intelligence.

The Cycle of Trigger and Response

Triggers often follow a predictable cycle:

1. **Stimulus**: Something external happens.
2. **Interpretation**: Your brain assigns meaning to it.
3. **Emotion**: You feel something intense—anger, fear, sadness, shame.
4. **Reaction**: You either explode, shut down, flee, or numb out.

To interrupt this cycle, insert a pause. That pause can be as small as three deep breaths. It can be a grounding phrase like, "This is familiar, but it's not the same." It can be the decision to journal before responding. That pause is where your power lives.

Emotional Recovery Plans

Just like you'd have a plan for a physical emergency, you need a recovery plan for emotional emergencies. Here's how you build one:

1. **Name your top triggers.** Be honest about what sends you spiraling.

2. **Identify your responses.** Do you shut down? Get defensive? Over-explain?
3. **List calming tools.** These could be grounding exercises, a walk, journaling, talking to someone safe, or repeating a comforting mantra.
4. **Write your "reset" script.** This is a short, kind message you can say to yourself in the moment: "I'm not broken. I'm just overwhelmed, and that's okay."
5. **Choose your safe space.** This could be a room, a person, a routine that feels anchoring. Go there when the emotional waves crash in.

What Not to Do After a Setback

- Don't shame yourself. Guilt will not help you heal faster.
- Don't isolate completely. Even if you need space, check in with someone who understands.
- Don't measure your worth by your worst moment.
- Don't compare your healing journey to anyone else's.

What to Do Instead

- Practice self-compassion. Talk to yourself like you would to a dear friend.
- Reflect on what happened without judgment.
- Use it as a learning opportunity.
- Celebrate your return to center, however long it takes.

Real-Life Examples

Maria had been managing her anxiety well for months. Then, during a family gathering, her uncle's comment about her weight triggered years of body shame. She spiraled into self-criticism. But instead of staying stuck, she went home, journaled her feelings, did a calming breathing exercise, and reminded herself: "My worth is not up for debate."

James, a teacher, prided himself on staying patient. But one afternoon, a student's disrespectful remark reminded him of how he used to be treated as a child. He snapped. Later, he apologized to the student, but more importantly, he forgave himself. He realized his reaction came from pain, not from who he is.

Your Long-Term Strategy

To deal with setbacks and triggers long-term, you need a combination of **self-awareness**, **tools**, and **support**. It's not about never being triggered again. It's about knowing what to do when it happens.

You can learn to:

- Notice the tension before it becomes an explosion
- Say "I need a moment" instead of saying something you regret
- Recognize patterns and shift them over time
- Show up for yourself with patience instead of punishment

Visual Anchor

Create a visual anchor for your healing journey.

Try this exercise: Draw a ladder with six steps. On each step, write what you can do when triggered, starting from most basic (e.g., "breathe deeply") to most advanced (e.g., "reframe my thoughts").

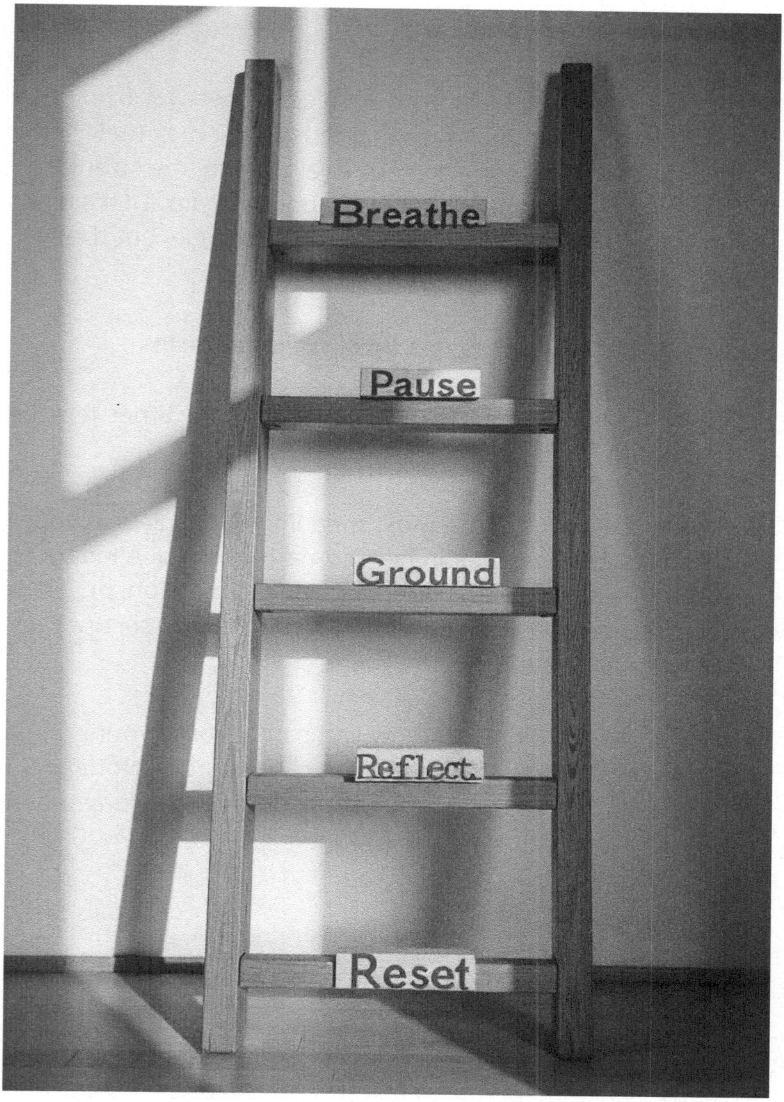
Breathe
Pause
Ground
Reflect.
Reset

Building Emotional Muscles

Every time you come back from a trigger or recover from a setback, you're building emotional muscles. It may feel like starting over, but you're not. You're reinforcing the strength to stand again, to regulate again, to choose again. That's what resilience looks like—not the absence of struggle, but the willingness to return.

Section 3: Turning Struggles Into Growth Stories

Pain is not the opposite of growth. In fact, many times it is the path to it.

When you look back at the most meaningful changes in your life, chances are, they began with something hard. A loss. A failure. A heartbreak. A season of waiting, confusion, or anxiety. Those were the moments you didn't choose, but they shaped who you became.

In this section, we'll explore how you can reframe your struggles not as detours, but as part of your story. Not as interruptions, but as the soil in which something stronger can grow.

Struggles Are Data, Not Definitions

It's easy to fall into the trap of defining ourselves by what broke us. "I'm someone who failed." "I'm the one who got left." "I'm the person who didn't make it."

But your pain is not your identity. It's an experience. And experiences are information.

Let's say you burnt out at your job. That's data.

It means something about your boundaries, your values, your workload, or even your beliefs about achievement might need some adjusting.

Or maybe you went through a messy breakup. That's data, too.

It tells you something about your needs, your patterns, your communication style, or your boundaries.

Struggles aren't a verdict. They're a signal. And when you shift your mindset from judgment to curiosity, you create the possibility for growth.

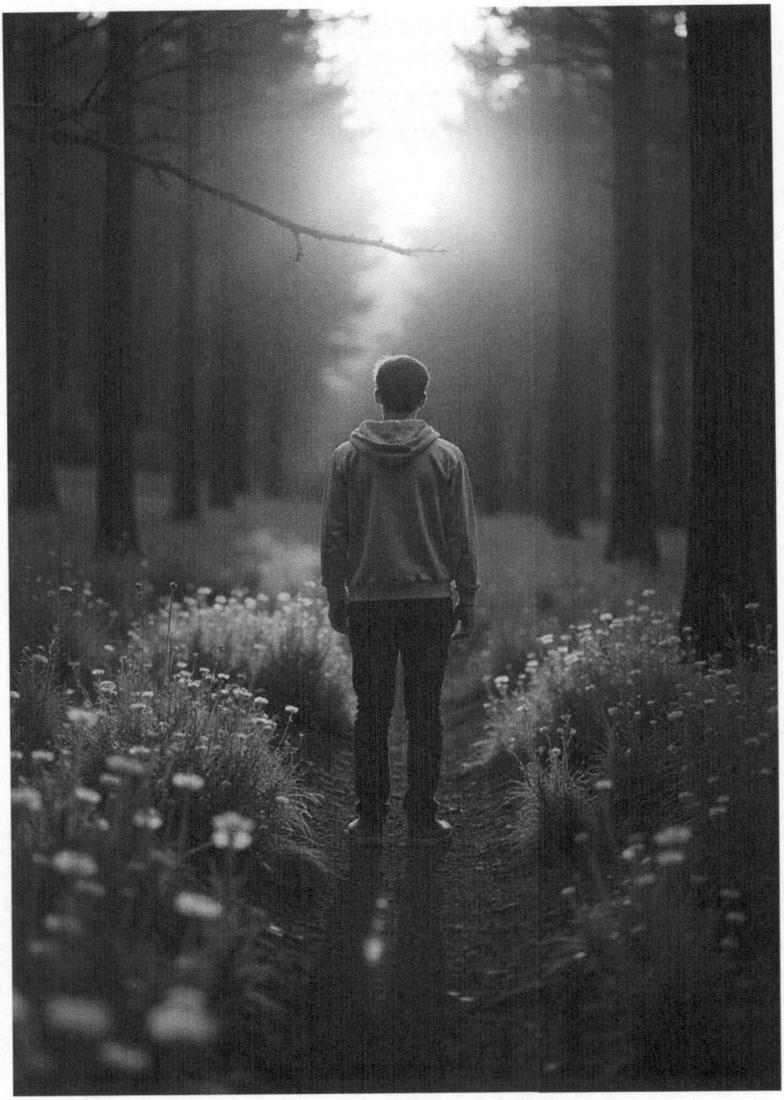

From Surviving to Storytelling

Have you ever heard someone tell their story of overcoming something, and felt hope rise in you?

The reason we love those stories is not because they were easy. It's because they were real. They had cracks and scars and turning points. They showed us that transformation isn't for perfect people—it's for people who kept going.

The invitation is not to wait until everything is resolved to begin telling your story. Start in the middle. Start with what you're learning.

You don't need to have the bow on top.

Growth stories are not linear. They are spiral-shaped. You come back to the same lessons with deeper understanding. You see progress, then backslide, then rise again.

The Power of Reframing

Reframing is the skill of taking a hard moment and asking, "What else could this mean?"

Instead of, "I failed," you might reframe: "I took a risk. That shows courage."

Instead of, "I'm broken," you might reframe: "I'm healing. That shows strength."

Reframing doesn't mean pretending everything is fine. It means you give yourself permission to see meaning *in* the mess.

Think of your life like a photo album. You get to choose which pictures to keep. Which captions to write. Which lessons to highlight. That's not denial. That's authorship.

Reframing your story doesn't erase the hard parts. It integrates them.

Using Your Struggles to Help Others

There is something sacred about using your pain to ease someone else's.

Whether it's through a conversation, a journal, a blog, or even just your presence, your story can be medicine.

You don't need a stage to be a storyteller. You just need to be honest.

Here are a few simple ways to share your growth:

- Write a letter to your past self and share what you've learned.
- Start a personal blog or social post where you document insights.
- Offer empathy, not advice, when someone else is struggling.
- Say, "Me too," instead of trying to fix someone's problem.

Note: You don't have to share everything. Protecting your privacy is an act of self-care. But sometimes, even the smallest piece of your journey can help someone else feel less alone.

The Beauty of Resilience

Resilience is not about bouncing back to who you were. It's about becoming someone wiser, softer, and stronger because of what you've faced.

Think of a tree that has grown crooked because of the wind. It might not look perfect, but it is *stronger* in the direction it had to grow.

You are that tree. And your resilience doesn't need applause. It already lives in your breath, your steps, your choices. Every time you get back up, even slowly, even silently, you are growing.

Turning Points Aren't Always Dramatic

Hollywood teaches us that big change always comes with thunder, epiphanies, and triumphant music. But real life is quieter.

A turning point can be:

- Saying no when you used to say yes.
- Getting out of bed when you wanted to give up.
- Starting therapy.
- Sending the text.
- Breathing instead of reacting.

These aren't small things. They're sacred things. Growth happens in the ordinary, and that's what makes it sustainable.

You don't need a miracle. You just need *one honest step* at a time.

Reflection: What Are You Growing Through?

Right now, ask yourself:

- What has been one of the hardest seasons of my life?
- What did I learn from it?
- How did it change me?
- What would I say to someone going through something similar?

These questions are not just about nostalgia. They're about clarity.

Every time you pause to reflect on your journey, you strengthen your sense of self. And that inner clarity becomes your compass when life throws you off course.

You Are Still Becoming

Your growth story isn't finished. But you are already so much more than you were.

You don't need to wait for a future version of yourself to start living with hope. You can start today, by honoring where you've been, embracing where you are, and leaning gently into what comes next.

You are not broken. You are becoming.

Section 4: Gratitude as a Daily Anchor

Gratitude is often underestimated. In a world that constantly chases the next big thing—a promotion, a purchase, a partner, or a perfectly balanced life—pausing to appreciate the present moment can feel both counterintuitive and revolutionary. But for anyone on a journey to lasting calm, emotional resilience, and personal growth, gratitude isn't just a nice idea. It is an essential tool, a daily anchor, and a mindset shift that quietly rewires the brain toward peace.

Let's explore how gratitude, practiced intentionally, can become your emotional compass. Not in a performative way, but as an honest, grounding force that helps you stay calm amid storms, hopeful during uncertainty, and connected to joy even when life is messy.

Gratitude Rewires the Brain for Calm

Science confirms what wisdom traditions have said for centuries: gratitude changes the way we experience the world. Neurological studies show that practicing gratitude activates the brain's reward centers and increases levels of dopamine and serotonin—our natural feel-good chemicals. Over time, gratitude actually rewires neural pathways, helping us to notice what's going well instead of fixating on what's wrong.

But what makes this tool so powerful isn't just its effects on mood; it's how gratitude gently pulls us away from stress-based reactivity. When you focus on what you're thankful for, your nervous system shifts from fight-or-flight into rest-and-digest mode. Gratitude helps regulate emotions, lower anxiety, and deepen your connection to the present.

In short, it calms the storm before it has a chance to build.

Daily Gratitude Isn't About Denial

Let's clear one thing up: gratitude doesn't mean denying your struggles. It doesn't ask you to ignore pain, pretend everything is okay, or slap on a smile. Real gratitude is not about sugar-coating reality. It's about learning to hold both joy and difficulty in the same hand.

You can grieve a loss and still feel grateful for the love you had. You can be overwhelmed and still be thankful for a moment of quiet. You can feel anxious about the future and still smile at the sun rising through your window. Gratitude, at its core, is about cultivating emotional flexibility.

It's the reminder that no matter how dark things get, there is always light somewhere—and that looking for it is not just healing but empowering.

The Micro-Moments of Gratitude

Gratitude doesn't have to be a grand gesture. You don't need to keep a thick journal filled with poetic reflections (unless you want to). It can be as simple as noting three things you're thankful for while brushing your teeth. It can be quietly saying thank you to your morning cup of tea, the warmth of your blanket, or the fact that you made it through the day.

Here are some practical ways to bring gratitude into your everyday life:

1. **Gratitude Bookends**: Begin and end your day by naming three things you're grateful for. Keep them simple. This creates a peaceful frame for your day.

2. **Sticky Note Reminders**: Place small gratitude reminders where you'll see them often—your mirror, laptop, fridge. Let them prompt you to pause and appreciate something.
3. **Gratitude Walks**: Go on a short walk and mentally list everything around you that sparks gratitude—sunlight, trees, birds, fresh air.
4. **Gratitude Jar**: Write one thing you're grateful for on a small piece of paper each day and drop it in a jar. At the end of the year (or during tough moments), read them back.
5. **Gratitude Text**: Once a week, send a simple thank-you text to someone who made your day brighter—a friend, colleague, or stranger.

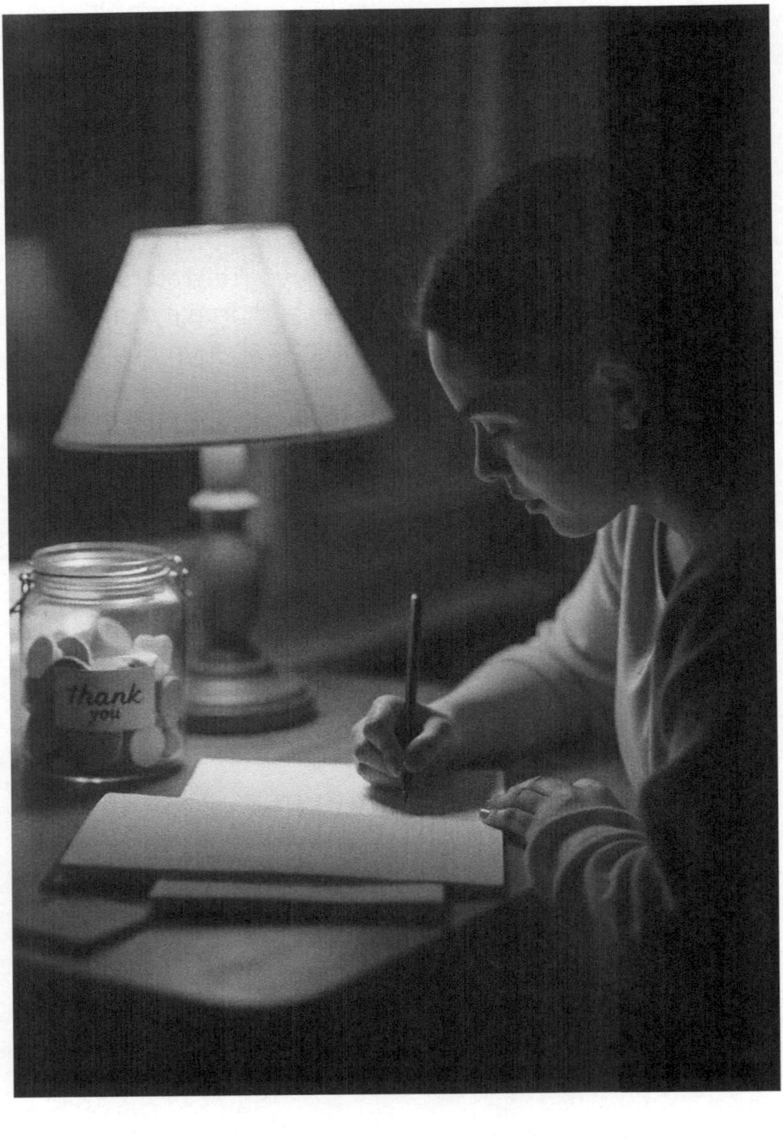
thank
you

Gratitude in Relationships

Gratitude strengthens not just your personal calm but your relationships too. When you regularly express appreciation to others—whether it's your partner, friend, parent, or child—it builds trust and deepens connection.

Studies show that couples who express gratitude regularly are more satisfied in their relationships. In workplaces, teams that acknowledge each other's efforts perform better and experience higher morale. Gratitude can disarm conflict, soften pride, and open the door to empathy.

Next time you're irritated with someone close to you, try shifting your focus: What do you appreciate about this person? What have they done, big or small, that you've taken for granted? Say it out loud. Watch what happens.

Gratitude in Crisis

During crises, gratitude may seem out of reach. But even in trauma recovery, gratitude has shown to support healing by providing a sense of meaning, strength, and coherence. Survivors of accidents, illness, loss, and war have shared how gratitude practices helped them feel anchored and hopeful.

This doesn't mean forcing positivity. But it does mean gently asking yourself: Is there anything, however small, that I can hold on to today? Gratitude doesn't eliminate the pain, but it gives you something else to look at besides your suffering.

Gratitude and Faith

For many, gratitude is a spiritual practice. In Christianity, for example, the Bible frequently urges believers to give thanks in all circumstances (1 Thessalonians 5:18). Not because everything is good, but because God is present through it all. Gratitude becomes a sacred dialogue, a way of remembering that we are not alone, even in hardship.

Whether your faith tradition is Christian or another, gratitude often forms a cornerstone of spiritual resilience. It roots you in a bigger story. It reminds you that there is more to your life than what hurts.

Building a Gratitude Habit

Making gratitude stick starts with intention. But it lasts with consistency. Here's how to build a habit that stays:

1. **Start Small**: Don't aim for perfection. Commit to 30 seconds a day.
2. **Pair It With Another Habit**: Tie your gratitude moment to brushing your teeth, morning coffee, or bedtime.
3. **Make It Visible**: Use a visual cue—a bracelet, a journal, a sticky note.
4. **Be Specific**: Instead of "I'm thankful for my family," say, "I'm grateful for the way my daughter laughed this morning."
5. **Reflect Regularly**: Revisit your gratitude notes at the end of the week to reinforce the practice.

Gratitude is not something you feel once and forget. It's a muscle that grows stronger with use. The more you practice it, the more you see the world through its lens.

Closing Thoughts: Gratitude is Not the End, It's the Beginning

When we talk about long-term calm, we're not aiming for a life without problems. We're creating a life with deeper roots. Gratitude is one of those roots. It grounds you. It whispers, "There is good here, too."

In many ways, gratitude is the beginning of emotional clarity, spiritual strength, and mental peace. It brings you back to what matters, over and over again. In a world that demands more, gratitude teaches you to say: "This is enough."

And when you can live from that place—from sufficiency, from stillness, from thanks—you become a calming force not just for yourself, but for others too.

Section 5: Surrounding Yourself With Uplifting Inputs

In a world where news cycles rarely rest, social media constantly buzzes, and negativity often dominates conversation, it becomes imperative to be intentional about what we consume. What you feed your mind is just as important as what you feed your body. In this section, we will explore how surrounding yourself with uplifting inputs — from people to podcasts, books to beliefs — can be a quiet but powerful form of self-care that sustains your resilience over the long term.

What Are "Uplifting Inputs"?

Think of uplifting inputs as anything that nourishes your mind, encourages your spirit, and elevates your perspective. This could be:

- Inspiring books that give hope
- Encouraging podcasts or uplifting music
- Conversations that energize instead of drain
- Nature, beauty, and silence
- Spiritual practices that align with your values

These are the emotional and mental equivalents of a balanced meal. Without them, we run the risk of being overloaded with junk — fear-based media, cynical commentary, and emotionally toxic voices.

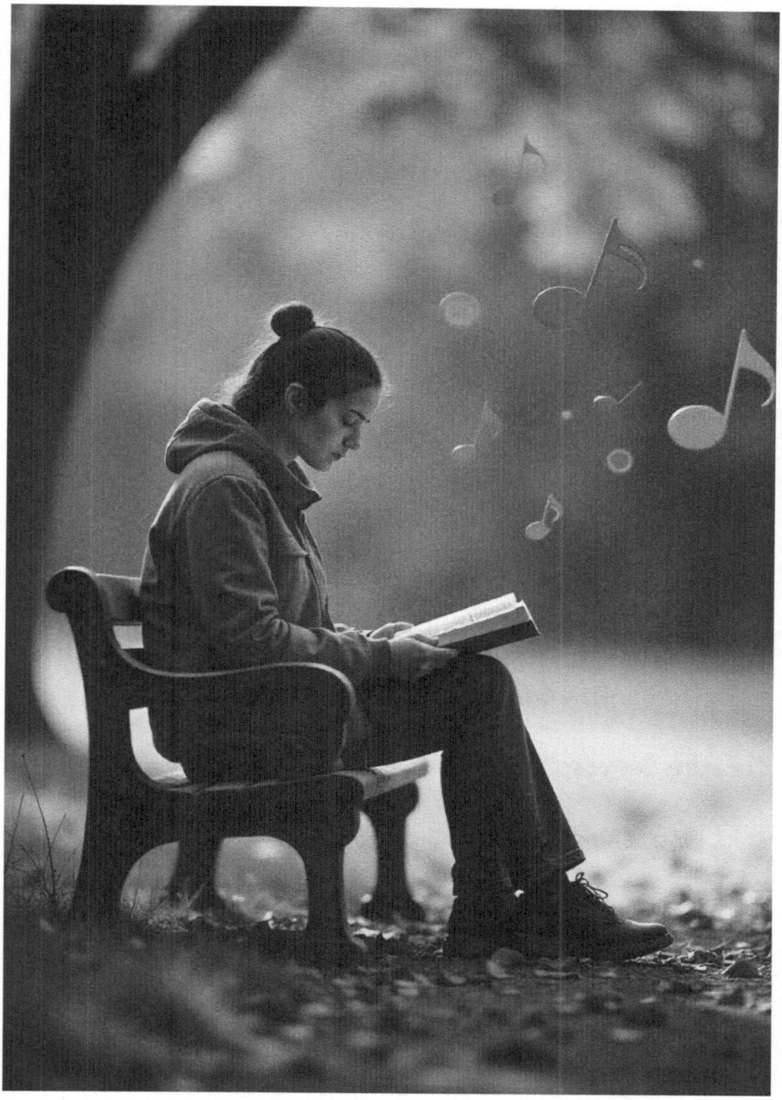

The Power of Input Overload

Many of us don't realize how much our daily inputs affect our thoughts, emotions, and even our behaviors. A single toxic news story in the morning can cast a shadow over our whole day. Scrolling through social media before bed can fill our minds with comparison, envy, or anxiety. Just as a garden choked with weeds struggles to grow flowers, a mind filled with unfiltered noise can struggle to stay hopeful.

Input Overload Symptoms:

- Constant worry or dread
- Feeling mentally drained without clear reason
- Reactivity or emotional numbness
- Difficulty focusing or sleeping

When these show up, it's often not a personal flaw — it's a sign that we need to audit what's going into our mental ecosystem.

Creating a Personal Input Audit

Start by tracking your emotional response to various inputs over the course of a week. Ask yourself:

- What do I listen to or watch first thing in the morning?
- How do I feel after spending time online?
- Are there certain people whose presence lifts or drains me?
- What media habits make me feel better vs. worse?

Jot these reflections down. Often, we don't even notice what's feeding us until we pause to reflect. Once you have awareness, you have power — the power to edit your input menu.

Choosing Inputs That Lift You Up

It doesn't require a total life overhaul to start feeding your spirit with better inputs. Here are some simple ways to do it:

1. Morning Routines with Intention

Replace the morning news with 10 minutes of peaceful music or an uplifting podcast. Start your day with a book that sparks your imagination instead of your anxiety.

2. Follow Hope, Not Hype

Be selective about your social media. Follow accounts that inspire you, educate you, or make you laugh without tearing others down. Unfollow or mute accounts that stir negative comparisons or fear.

3. Surround Yourself With Uplifting People

Energy is contagious. Spend time with people who reflect the values you want to grow. Seek those who are honest but hopeful, grounded but growth-minded. Even a short conversation with the right person can reset your entire mindset.

4. Create a "Joy Shelf"

Dedicate a physical or digital space to your favorite uplifting things. A shelf of books that always restore you. A playlist that never fails to lift your mood. A folder of encouraging notes, screenshots, or quotes.

The Impact of Nature and Stillness

Not all inputs are digital or social. Nature is one of the most underrated sources of calm and resilience. Walking in a park, tending to plants, or simply watching the clouds can reduce cortisol and boost your mood.

Silence is another powerful input. In a noisy world, choosing moments of intentional quiet helps you hear your inner voice more clearly. Schedule moments of digital detox, where you unplug to reconnect with yourself.

Don't Ignore the Subtle Voices

Sometimes the most uplifting inputs aren't grand gestures but tiny, quiet things that whisper peace:

- A cup of tea made slowly and mindfully
- A kind message sent or received
- A verse or phrase repeated as an anchor
- The sound of birds or rain

These are the sacred pauses in our day that offer deep rest for the soul.

What If You Live in a Toxic Environment?

You might not have full control over your surroundings — maybe your workplace is high-stress, or your family dynamics are complicated. But even in difficult spaces, you can curate micro-moments of peace:

- Use headphones to play calming music while you work
- Keep a quote card or calming image in your pocket

- Step outside for a few breaths of fresh air whenever possible

You have more power than you think to inject light into dark spaces. It begins with intention.

Building Your Input Circle: A Sample Plan

Try this weekly rhythm to keep your uplifting inputs balanced:

Monday:

- 10 minutes of journaling gratitude before work
- Uplifting podcast during commute

Tuesday:

- Digital detox during lunch hour
- Inspirational TED Talk before bed

Wednesday:

- Walk in nature
- Chat with a positive friend

Thursday:

- Read a chapter from a calming or inspiring book

Friday:

- End the week by reflecting on small wins
- Share a kind word with someone else

Weekend:

- Attend a spiritual gathering or quiet reflection
- Watch a feel-good movie or cook a favorite meal

This isn't about perfection but intention. Think of it as tending your internal garden. Some days you water it fully. Other days, a single sunbeam is enough.

Final Reflection

Just like food, what you consume emotionally and mentally will either drain you or build you. By choosing uplifting inputs with intention, you're not escaping reality — you're equipping yourself to face it with greater strength.

Your peace is precious. Guard it not with walls, but with wisdom.

Section 6: Living Intentionally: Small Wins, Big Peace

There's a quiet kind of power that lives in the everyday. Not in the applause, not in the milestones—but in those tiny, often invisible moments where we choose to be mindful, gentle, and real. This is what living intentionally is about. It's not about having a perfectly scheduled life or checking off a thousand goals. It's about pausing long enough to ask, "What matters most today?" and then showing up for that answer with grace.

What Is Intentional Living?

Intentional living means aligning your actions with your values. It means choosing your response rather than reacting impulsively. It's about creating a life on purpose—not by default. For someone navigating anxiety or emotional burnout, this shift in approach can be healing. Instead of always trying to control outcomes, you begin to honor your inner compass.

It's in waking up and drinking your coffee slowly, instead of scrolling your phone. It's in choosing to take the longer walk home because you need the silence. It's in saying no to a social gathering because you're building boundaries. These seemingly small decisions accumulate and pave the way for a grounded, resilient life.

Small Wins Matter More Than We Think

We often chase the idea that progress only counts if it's dramatic. But the truth? Big peace comes from small wins. That's how habits are built, how healing becomes sustainable, and how calm starts to settle in like a familiar rhythm.

Here are a few examples of small wins:

- Taking five minutes to breathe before responding to a stressful email.
- Drinking a glass of water first thing in the morning.
- Saying, "I need a moment" instead of pretending you're okay.
- Cleaning a single drawer when everything else feels overwhelming.
- Journaling one sentence about how you feel.

These things might seem insignificant—but they represent intentionality. They say: *"I matter enough to pause and care for myself, even in small ways."*

The Power of a Daily Reset

Living intentionally doesn't mean you never get overwhelmed. It means you create systems to return to center when you do. Daily resets are one of the best tools for this.

A reset might be as simple as:

- Taking a ten-minute walk to clear your mind.
- Lighting a candle and practicing five deep breaths.
- Turning off notifications for an hour.
- Changing into comfy clothes and stretching.

These resets recalibrate your nervous system. They're like hitting "refresh" on your day. With consistency, you teach your brain that peace is accessible—even on hard days.

Morning and Evening Anchors

Two of the most powerful places to add intentionality? The beginning and end of your day. These moments bookend your emotional energy.

Morning anchors might include:

- Waking up without immediately reaching for your phone.
- Taking 3-5 minutes to journal your intentions for the day.
- Saying a quiet prayer or affirmation: *"I choose peace today."*

Evening anchors might include:

- Reflecting on one thing you're grateful for.

- Releasing the day's tension through breathing exercises.
- Reading or listening to something that calms your mind.

These rituals don't have to be long or complex. What matters is that they're yours. Consistency turns them into a safe container for your emotions.

Letting Go of Perfection

Intentional living is not another perfectionistic trap. You don't have to live every moment "mindfully" or never mess up. The goal is not flawless peace—it's self-awareness. There will be days when you're reactive, days when you spiral, and days when you forget every tool you've learned.

The win isn't in never falling off track. It's in noticing and returning gently. In saying, *"Today was hard, but tomorrow I try again."*

This compassionate mindset keeps you out of shame and keeps you moving forward.

Saying No to Make Space for Yes

One of the most overlooked parts of intentional living is subtraction. Sometimes peace isn't found by adding more affirmations or meditations—but by removing the things that crowd your mental and emotional space.

This could mean:

- Muting toxic social media accounts.
- Unsubscribing from email lists that cause pressure.
- Releasing relationships that drain you.

- Quitting commitments that no longer align.

By saying no to what doesn't align, you make room to say yes to the life you want to create.

Celebrate the Wins — Even If They're Quiet

Intentional living is deeply personal. It won't always make sense to others. You may not get applause for choosing rest over hustle. But the peace you gain? That's your reward.

Celebrate your quiet victories:

- When you choose to respond kindly to yourself.
- When you slow down even though the world is speeding up.
- When you listen to your body and rest.

Each small win sends a message to your soul: *"I am safe. I am worthy. I am enough."*

Summary of Chapter 8: The Long Game — Living With Resilience and Hope

This chapter is about sustainable peace. Not the fleeting kind that only exists when life is calm, but the deep kind that roots itself in daily decisions. Here's what we've explored:

1. **Long-Term Calm** is a way of being, not a final destination. It's how you move through the world—grounded, compassionate, and in sync with your values.

2. **Setbacks and Emotional Triggers** are not signs of failure. They are part of the process. Learning how to respond rather than react is a powerful shift.
3. **Your Struggles Can Become Growth Stories**. The hard things shape your wisdom. You are not your pain—but you are more resilient because of it.
4. **Gratitude** is a daily anchor that can transform even the hardest seasons. It rewires your brain for peace and presence.
5. **Uplifting Inputs** matter. What you consume becomes how you feel. Curate your surroundings with care.
6. **Intentional Living** teaches you that small wins—like a deep breath, a kind word, a five-minute break—are what build a peaceful, hopeful life.

Peace isn't just something you reach. It's something you *live*. Not every day will be easy, but every day offers the opportunity to return to yourself, one gentle, intentional step at a time.

You don't need to become someone else. You don't need to chase a perfect version of calm. You simply need to become more *you*—kind, intentional, and grounded.

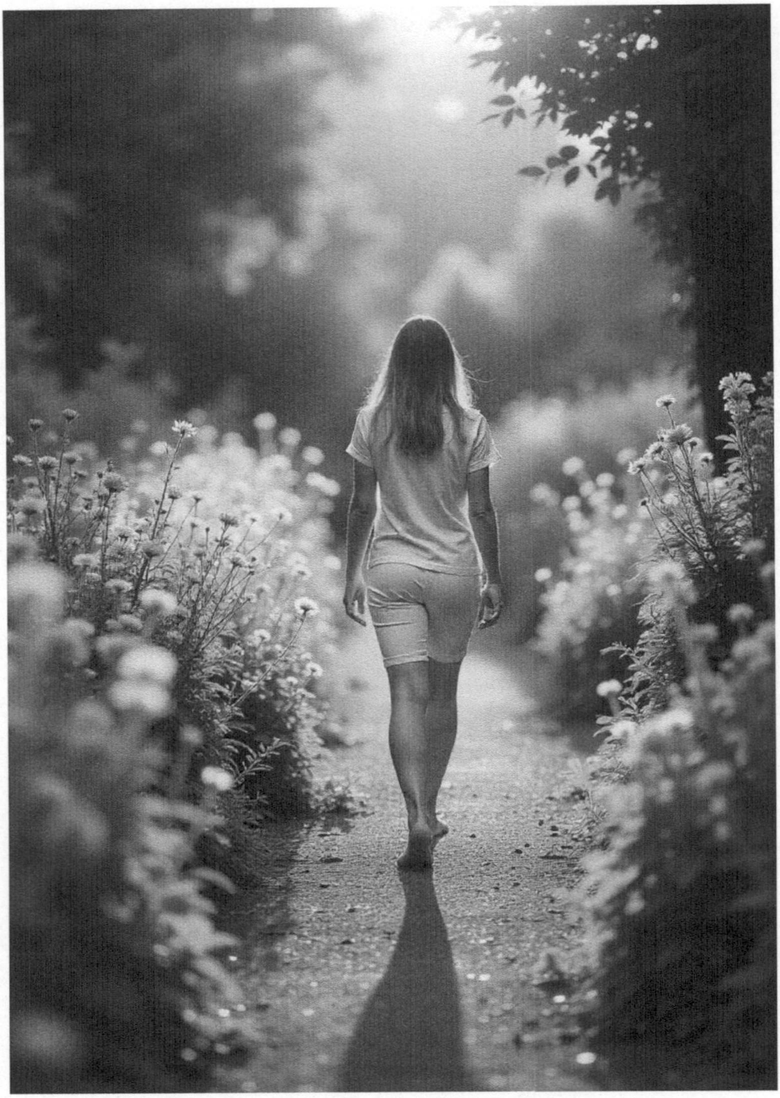

Conclusion: Your Calm is Not a Luxury — It's a Right

You Don't Have to Be "Fixed" to Be Free

Take a deep breath. Let that sink in.

The calm you seek is not a reward for being perfect. It isn't a prize for healing fast enough or getting life right on the first try. It doesn't arrive only when the world outside is quiet. It can exist in you now—right now. Not because you've done everything right, but simply because you're human, and you deserve peace.

In a world constantly shouting that we must hustle, fix ourselves, change, upgrade, and never stop grinding, choosing calm feels like a rebellion. But it's a necessary one. You don't have to earn your calm. It is your birthright.

Peace isn't something far away or something only the "zen" people find in mountaintop retreats. It's not a luxury item to be unlocked after productivity. It is something you can access in everyday life—even if your house is messy, your inbox is full, your body is tired, and your heart is still healing.

One Step a Day Is Enough

Maybe after reading this book, you're feeling inspired—but also overwhelmed. You might be thinking: "There's so much I want to change. Where do I start?"

The truth is, you don't have to do it all at once.

One small step today is more powerful than a grand plan you never start. The key is consistency, not intensity. Maybe today, that one step is drinking water slowly. Maybe it's saying no without apologizing. Maybe it's journaling one sentence before bed. These are not small things. They are sacred.

We live in a culture obsessed with dramatic transformation. But the most profound changes often come quietly, in the decisions we make every day to show up differently for ourselves.

"I will pause before I react."

"I will choose what nourishes me, not just what is expected of me."

"I will rest without guilt."

These are your milestones. These are your victories.

Over time, these daily practices compound. And before you realize it, you are living a calmer, clearer, more resilient life—not because you became someone else, but because you honored who you already are.

Let This Book Be the Beginning

This book wasn't written as a solution. It's not a checklist. It's a doorway.

What comes next is yours to shape.

Maybe you'll revisit a chapter when a hard day hits. Maybe you'll create your own Calm Toolkit and update it every season. Maybe you'll start noticing when your breath gets shallow and choose to deepen it instead.

You now have the tools to:

- Recognize your own anxiety signals
- Set healthy, compassionate boundaries
- Create space in your day for rest and recovery
- Handle difficult conversations with clarity
- Learn to reset when things go wrong
- And most importantly, to trust yourself again

This journey is ongoing, and that's the beauty of it. You're allowed to keep learning, stumbling, recalibrating. You're allowed to grow slowly. Progress isn't always linear. Sometimes peace shows up in the middle of the mess.

So when life gets loud again (and it will), you don't need to panic. You have options. You have yourself.

A Personal Letter from the Author

Dear Reader,

If you made it here, know this: I'm proud of you.

Not for finishing this book (though that's a big deal!), but for choosing to care about your peace. For choosing, in a world full of noise, to listen inward.

I didn't write this book because I figured life out. I wrote it because I needed it. There were years when calm felt like a foreign land, and my thoughts were a storm I couldn't outrun. I searched for answers in books, podcasts, conversations, and late-night journaling sessions—only to realize that the answers were always within. They were just waiting for space.

Maybe you see yourself in that story.

If you take one thing away from this book, let it be this: You are not broken. You are becoming. And calm is not reserved for the few—it's a daily invitation for all.

I hope this book has helped you name your needs, soften your inner voice, and return home to yourself. I hope it made you feel less alone. I hope you know, now more than ever, that you are worthy of peace without performing for it.

This is not the end.

It's just the next breath.

With deep gratitude and hope,

Enoch Merlyn

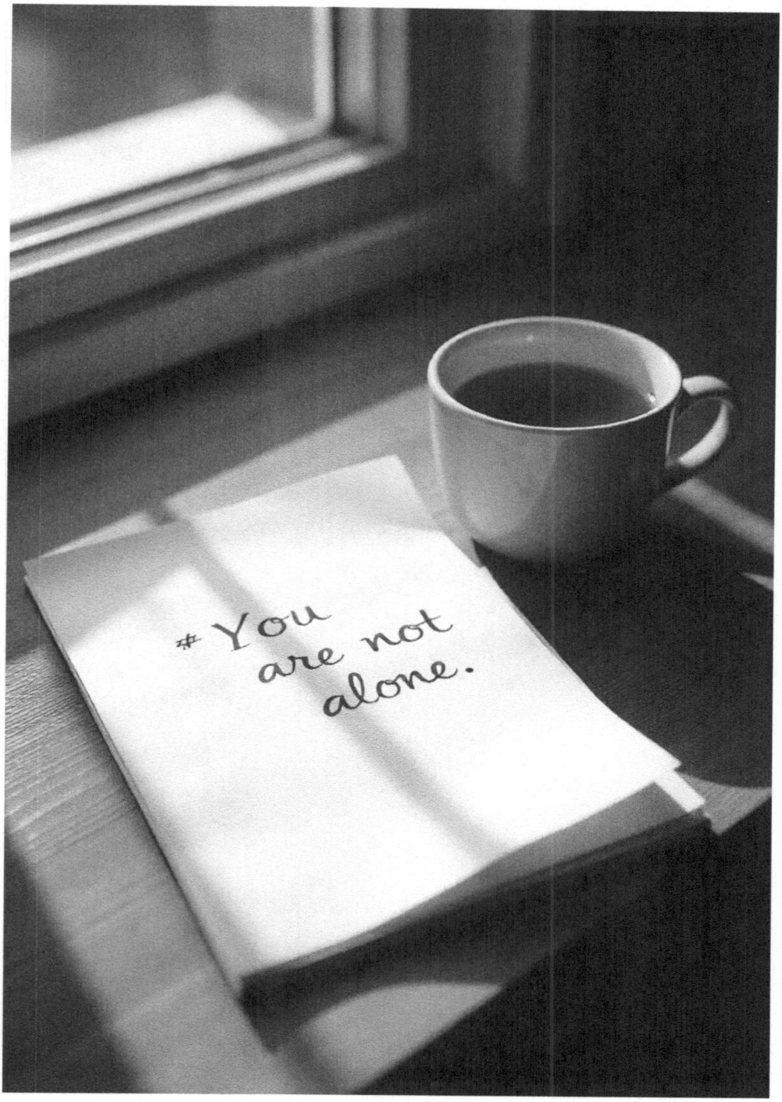

* You
are not
alone.

Final Reflection: A Gentle Reminder

Before you close this book, take one last moment to pause.

Ask yourself:

- What has shifted in me while reading?
- What is one gentle action I can take today?
- How can I be kinder to myself going forward?

Then breathe. Smile if you can. You're doing better than you think.

The journey to peace isn't about rushing to the end. It's about learning to stay with yourself along the way.

Welcome home.

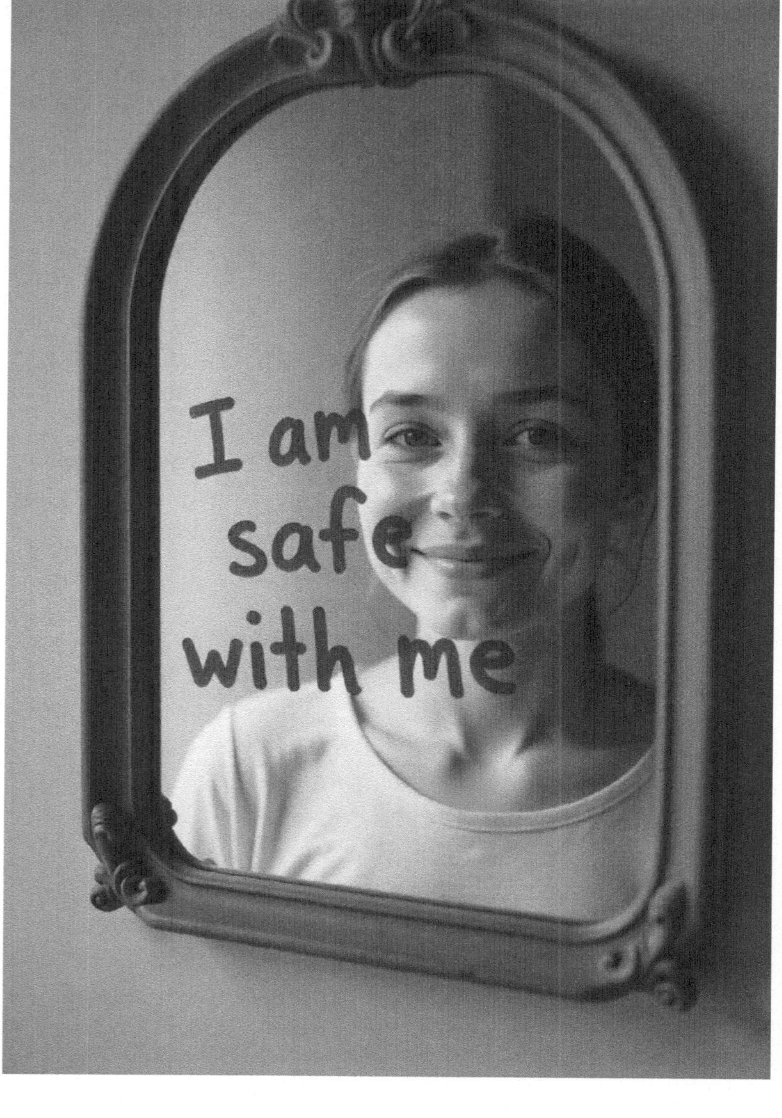
I am
safe
with me

About the Author

Enoch Merlyn is an experienced professional with over 28 years of diverse industry expertise — including more than 17 years in the IT sector, where he continues to work today. His extensive journey through sales, technical service, entrepreneurship, and technology has given him a unique lens on personal growth, resilience, and real-world problem-solving.

From his early days selling telecom equipment and training service teams, to leading customer support in the electronics and security systems sectors, Enoch's career has always centered around helping people — whether through service, mentorship, or leadership. Now, in the ever-evolving world of information technology, he brings the same mindset to empowering others through his writing.

He holds a Diploma in Electronics and Communication Engineering and a Bachelor's degree in Computer Applications. His combined technical knowledge and people-first experience make him especially skilled at translating complex ideas into simple, practical strategies for everyday life — a hallmark of his self-help books.

As a devoted husband and proud father to a child with autism, Enoch understands life's challenges on a deeply personal level. His writing is shaped by compassion, discipline, and a desire to support others who are seeking clarity, calm, and personal transformation.

A lifelong learner and passionate reader, he draws inspiration from global authors and beloved Tamil writers such as Sujatha and Balakumaran. Through his books, Enoch Merlyn helps readers take small, actionable steps toward building better habits, stronger mindsets, and more meaningful lives.

Enjoyed the book? Share your thoughts! □ □ □ □ □

Your feedback means the world! Leave a quick review and let others know how this book helped you.

Want Free Bonus Resources?
Take your calm journey deeper with these FREE, beautifully designed tools:

7-Day Calm Reset Challenge
Your Personal Calm Toolkit Printable
Anxious to Anchored: Daily Journal Template
The Anxious Generation Self-Test + Reflection Guide

Just send a quick email to: **EnochMerlyn@gmail.com**
with the subject **"Send My Calm Tools"** — and I'll personally email them to you!

Thank you for your support!

References

1. American Psychological Association. (2023). *Stress in America™ Survey*. Retrieved from www.apa.org
2. Brach, T. (2003). *Radical Acceptance: Embracing Your Life With the Heart of a Buddha*. Bantam.
3. Brown, B. (2010). *The Gifts of Imperfection: Let Go of Who You Think You're Supposed to Be and Embrace Who You Are*. Hazelden Publishing.
4. Center for Mindful Self-Compassion. (n.d.). *Research Support for MSC*. Retrieved from https://centerformsc.org
5. Chodron, P. (2002). *When Things Fall Apart: Heart Advice for Difficult Times*. Shambhala Publications.
6. Davidson, R. J., & Begley, S. (2012). *The Emotional Life of Your Brain*. Penguin.
7. Harris, R. (2008). *The Happiness Trap: How to Stop Struggling and Start Living*. Trumpeter.
8. Kabat-Zinn, J. (1990). *Full Catastrophe Living: Using the Wisdom of Your Body and Mind to Face Stress, Pain, and Illness*. Delacorte.
9. Linehan, M. M. (1993). *Skills Training Manual for Treating Borderline Personality Disorder*. Guilford Press. *(Referenced for DBT skills such as grounding, emotion regulation, and distress tolerance.)*
10. Neff, K. (2011). *Self-Compassion: The Proven Power of Being Kind to Yourself*. William Morrow.
11. Porges, S. W. (2011). *The Polyvagal Theory: Neurophysiological Foundations of Emotions, Attachment, Communication, and Self-Regulation*. Norton.
12. Siegel, D. J. (2010). *The Mindful Therapist: A Clinician's Guide to Mindsight and Neural Integration*. W. W. Norton & Company.
13. van der Kolk, B. (2014). *The Body Keeps the Score: Brain, Mind, and Body in the Healing of Trauma*. Viking.

14. World Health Organization. (2022). *Mental health: Strengthening our response*. Retrieved from www.who.int
15. Young, K. S. (2009). *Cognitive Behavioral Therapy for Anxiety and Depression*. American Psychological Association.

9 789334 425055

Printed at Repro India Ltd.